Amanda
Ellison

Splitting

The Inside Story
on Headaches

GREEN TREE
LONDON · OXFORD · NEW YORK · NEW DELHI · SYDNEY

GREEN TREE
Bloomsbury Publishing Plc
50 Bedford Square, London, WC1B 3DP, UK

BLOOMSBURY, GREEN TREE and the Green Tree logo are trademarks
of Bloomsbury Publishing Plc

First published in Great Britain 2020

A catalogue record for this book is available from the British Library

Library of Congress Cataloguing-in-Publication data has been applied for

ISBN: HB: 978-1-4729-7141-8; PB: 978-1-4729-7140-1; eBook:978-1-4729-7144-9;
ePdf: 978-1-4729-7143-2

2 4 6 8 10 9 7 5 3 1

Typeset in Baskerville by Deanta Global Publishing Services, Chennai, India
Printed and bound in Great Britain by CPI Group (UK) Ltd, Croydon CR0 4YY

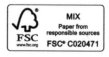

Bloomsbury Publishing Plc makes every effort to ensure that the papers used in the manufacture
of our books are natural, recyclable products made from wood grown in well-managed forests.
Our manufacturing processes conform to the environmental regulations of the country of origin.

To find out more about our authors and books visit www.bloomsbury.com
and sign up for our newsletters

For my Mum and Dad: Mary and Aidan Ellison.
Always, forever, love and thanks.

Contents

1

And So It Begins

WE'VE ALL HAD THAT uh-oh feeling. Something doesn't feel quite right. There's a tightness, a fogginess, a malaise, a pain. Thirty minutes later we might use other words: splitting, pounding, banging. Now it's a headache.

This happened to me recently. I was late for a meeting and I couldn't find my glasses. I have pretty good vision, my ophthalmologist tells me, except my left eye is shaped like a rugby ball instead of a soccer ball so I see the world on a bit of a slant. It doesn't make much of a difference to my everyday life since my brain compensates really well. However, if I am tired and working on a computer, my brain doesn't have to work so hard if I have a corrective lens. On this particular day, I was very tired. I had made the mistake of watching a dystopian drama the previous night with a glass of wine, and I couldn't get to sleep. The last time I looked at the clock it was 3.13 a.m. I knew I'd need my glasses; just looking at things seemed effortful. I had an hour-long drive to get to my meeting and every minute I spent looking for my specs diminished the likelihood I would find a parking spot near where I was going, guaranteeing a sprint to the venue on the other end. And I do not sprint.

Despite my frantic search, I didn't find my glasses before I had to go. I parked a 15-minute hustle from the meeting I was 10 minutes late for. Although I hate tardiness, everybody was very understanding and the meeting only really started when I got there in my slightly hot and bothered state. Work was done, progress was made, although the meeting ran long. I seemed to chase my tail all day. By the time I got home at 6 p.m. all I wanted for dinner was a paracetamol sandwich. Why? Because my head felt like it was in the grip of giant hands and they had begun to squeeze.

We need pain. It seems contradictory to say it, particularly now that we have so many ways of dealing with it and switching it off, but pain not only tells us that something is wrong, but it also protects us. If you slam the car door on your hand, it's going to hurt like Hades. You will have damaged the soft tissue, all the muscles and ligaments that help you move your fingers. It will no doubt swell up to twice its size, making it hard to move anyway. This inflammation is part of the healing process. The blood vessels in your hand get bigger, dilating to bring more blood containing all of the things the body needs to repair itself; mast cells that release histamine (*see* p. 26), which helps the blood vessels become more leaky, allowing white blood cells and proteins into the damaged area to protect and fix what's broken. (Prostaglandins are inflammatory hormones found all over your body that do this too.) Your hand feels hot and looks red because of all the extra blood flow and it throbs like crazy, maybe to the beat of your heart. All of these inflammatory agents that are acting to heal you are stimulating the pain receptors in your hand, the ones in your skin and your muscles. Every time you move your hand it hurts even more. So, as your doctor might say, don't move it, at least not initially. Every time you do, you stop the repair work and probably undo some of the progress that has been made. Pain tells you not to move it. Eventually, though, the pain becomes less paralysing, allowing you to get some mobility back.

Your head is not much different, although it is highly unusual to slam your head in a car door. The main difference is that the underlying cause of your hurting head can be much more subtle and varied. I can point to many reasons for my headache last week. Stress is the obvious one, eye strain is another. I missed lunch because everything was delayed and I am pretty sure I didn't hydrate well. Couple this with the tiredness I was experiencing because of my lack of sleep, which could have been related to the alcohol I had drunk or the rubbish I had watched on the television the previous night, and it is clear that I had precipitated the perfect storm in my skull. The pain that I was feeling was coming from the blood vessels in my head – the ones that feed my brain; this cerebrovascular system, as the blood vessels are known, brings glucose (which is the only fuel the brain can use), oxygen and other nutrients to the brain, but it doesn't mix with all the nerves and other cells that live there. In fact, blood is toxic to the brain, which is why it's kept separate from the brain tissue through the blood brain barrier. Therefore, if the blood vessels of the cerebrovascular system dilate for any reason, alarm bells ring in the form of pain to signal this risk to you.

The typical brain weighs about 1.4kg (3lb) and is made up of nerve cells – neurons – of different types, and the cells that support these neurons. It works through a balance of specific parts for specific functions all communicating to bring about the seamless transition between taking in and understanding everything that our senses tell us and us then reacting to them. For example, to pick up a spoon, you first have to see it (engaging the visual occipital regions at the back of the brain), recognise it (which involves the temporal cortex above your ear), remember what you do with the spoon (using the parietal cortex towards the top of your head behind the midline) and send the commands to your hand to pick it up and use it (engaging the front of your brain) to eat the ice cream you have been craving (thank you, hypothalamus).

The brain works under tight parameters, and as you use various bits of it, blood flow is diverted there to give that part the energy it needs to function. So, thinking and problem solving will mean that blood flow is diverted to your frontal lobe, whereas working your visual system diverts flow to your occipital regions. Pain happens when there is a breakdown between what your brain needs and what your vascular system, which carries your blood around, can bring it. If your visual system needs to work harder because you forgot to wear your glasses, more and more blood will be diverted there to help you cope. If perhaps you didn't eat so well during the day, the blood won't have as much glucose in it as it should, so even more blood is diverted to the visual system to provide the energy it requires. All the blood vessels get bigger or dilate – a process called 'vasodilation' – to bring more blood quickly and this stretches their walls beyond comfortable limits, setting off the pain receptors in your blood vessels. 'There is danger here', is their message, 'stop what you are doing'.

Depending on the type of headache, the pain will cleverly change our behaviour, sometimes incapacitating us – as is the case with cluster headache and migraine – allowing our blood vessels to get back to normal without any further stress or distraction.

Now, it is very unlikely that blood vessels will actually burst in reaction to a taxing day like the one I described, particularly since I don't have a heart condition or history of fainting and am not elderly, yet. However, headache is not to be taken lightly, particularly if you play contact sports or if it comes on suddenly, or you wake up with it, or if it is accompanied by speech, vision or movement problems. Any of these may indicate that a blood vessel has burst and has damaged brain tissue, or that you have a blockage to a blood vessel that is starving the brain of nutrients. Bear in mind that these causes of headache are no respecters of age; stroke is more common in the elderly because the elasticity of the blood vessels diminishes as we get older, meaning they are less able to cope with dilation and contraction, while younger people can suffer malformations in the cerebrovascular system, known as aneurysms, whereby bulbs can form in a previously tubular blood vessel.

Pill popping

Painkillers help ease headaches and the associated pain, as their name suggests. Simple over-the-counter medications like paracetamol (from para-aceto-amino-phenol or acetaminophen in America) and ibuprofen decrease the inflammation and help the blood vessels get back to a normal width so that they stop tugging on the pain receptors embedded in their walls. However, you may be surprised to learn that overusing these drugs for every ache and pain can actually lead to headache itself. They act to constrict all blood vessels, not just the ones where you might be

Aneurysms

An aneurysm (from the Greek for 'dilation' or 'widening') is a bulge in a blood vessel that can happen most commonly in the brain or the abdomen. Because of the bulge, blood doesn't flow down the vessel as it should, instead going into the bulge and coming out again in a turbulent way. Because the vessel wall that has bulged is weakened, there is the risk that the little balloon it has made will burst, and so it will cause a bleed on the brain. Most aneurysms go undetected until they actually rupture, but sometimes they are spotted if doctors are looking for something else. The good news is that once a specialist knows it is there, its growth can be monitored, and together, neurosurgeon and patient can decide whether to just watch it and wait or do something about it with surgery.

If it does rupture, the headache that results from a bleed on the brain, or subarachnoid haemorrhage, is described as sudden and agonising – the worst headache you have ever experienced. You may also have a stiff neck, a severe aversion to light and sickness or nausea. Some of these symptoms are shared with migraine, given that the pain pathway is the same, but with bleeding on the brain you have triggered all sorts of alarm systems to tell you something is wrong as blood is toxic to brain tissue and kills it on contact. And so with a haemorrhage, symptoms are more diffuse, with more clinical features. Either way, it is never wise to ignore a type of headache you have never experienced before. Always see your medical professional; it could save your life.

feeling the pain, so if you use them for more than 15 days per month for three months, the cerebrovascular system has to constantly readjust to keep blood flow regular to the brain (which is of paramount importance), and this can break down, leading to headache. This side effect of painkiller usage is most important for those suffering from chronic pain disorders such as arthritis and is why other treatments, such as movement therapy, are important, particularly when the condition first presents itself.

Nevertheless, occasionally taking over-the-counter medications can help, especially if they are used alongside caffeine. This is because caffeine also causes blood vessels to constrict, which is what painkillers do. In addition, it can help the absorption of paracetamol through the digestive system. Indeed, it often comes in the same tablet in many over-the-counter medications for pain. It has also been reported in scientific journals that Coca-Cola can increase the absorption of ibuprofen to such an extent that you may not need to take as much ibuprofen to feel the same pain relief!

More heavy-duty painkillers such as morphine act on the brain's *perception* of pain (as opposed to stopping the inflammation that causes the pain) by mimicking the natural painkillers, or endorphins, that exist in the body. You can buy a form of morphine called codeine from the pharmacy, often packaged with paracetamol. Morphine doesn't lend itself to tablet form because it doesn't get absorbed through the gut; the most effective way to take it is directly, by injection. Codeine, however, is a precursor to morphine that can be broken down in the liver by an enzyme called CY2PD6 into morphine, which then acts to damp down or stop the pain signals getting to our conscious brain.

Interestingly, 10 per cent of us don't have this enzyme and so we can't break down codeine, making it relatively useless to us. We may as well be eating sweets! (Or might I suggest chocolate, which contains a precursor to our happy hormone, serotonin.) In fact, we all have different levels of natural endorphins, and this is what determines our natural pain thresholds; a high concentration means you might be able to cope calmly with slamming your hand in your car door, whereas the same action may make someone else scream expletives in pain, perhaps indicating that they have lower endorphin levels. (Although as studies have shown, cursing *can* actually help boost natural painkilling action, though not if you are a potty mouth to begin with.)

Water as medicine

Before you reach for the painkillers, effective in the short term as they may be, it is worth understanding where your headache comes from to make sure you are fixing it once and for all, and to do this you need to learn about hydration. The most common fix for minor nagging headache comes out of your tap.

The human form is merely a bag, of which 60 per cent is taken up with water. Every cell in your body contains water, and so does the fluid that surrounds your cells. Clearly, it is important stuff. And yet we lose water every second of the day. We breathe it out, we use it to moisten the air we breathe in, we use it to dilute the toxins our body produces in order to safely wee them out. We sweat water out through our skin. We also use it to digest our food and it is involved in the formation of our stools, making them soft enough to be expelled comfortably.

The hypothalamus, which you will soon discover is my favourite part of the brain, controls how much water we have in our systems; it drives our thirst, making us drink liquids. Water is obviously best, but most people drink other things, too, which we need to dilute in our kidneys in order to excrete them safely – things like coffee, tea and alcohol. These are diuretics, which means that they make us urinate more, sometimes causing us to lose more water than the drink provided us with in the first place.

If we don't have enough water in our bloodstream to dilute the toxins in our kidneys then we become dehydrated. This is because the kidneys will take water from wherever they can in the body, regardless of how much it may be needed elsewhere. Your brain contains a whopping 1.4 litres (2½ pints) of water – a veritable oasis that can be tapped in times of crisis. So, this is where a good proportion of that water your kidneys need comes from if you haven't been drinking enough, causing your brain to literally shrink in the process, like a dry sponge.

This shrinking is the cause of the most common headache – a dehydration headache – whereby the whole brain pulls on the covering of the brain, the meninges ('men-in-gees' – from the Greek *mēning* for 'membrane') activating its pain receptors. Commonly recognised as the 'hangover headache' because alcohol is a prolific dehydrator, it really can happen at any time if we are not hydrating properly – something that is all too easy to do, especially if it is warm and we are sweating a lot. You get the picture. Water matters. Taking a painkiller helps to dull the pain but in this case it doesn't address the underlying problem: our brain needs water, and only when that has been replenished will the pain signals stop.

Your brain and your behaviour

Our headaches are therefore born as much from our behaviours – what we eat, what we drink, what we do when we are busy or stressed – as what is going on inside our heads and what we ask our brains to do. For example, thinking is the most fun that you can have on your own, but overthinking can make your brain hurt, right? Well, it's not your brain itself that hurts – in fact the cerebral cortex, made famous in pictures of the human brain the world over, is the only place in your body that doesn't have any sensory or pain receptors – but your brain does translate the signals coming from the blood vessels in your head as pain if they are overstretched, or if your body is having to work too hard to get the right amount of blood to your brain to help you think.

In the chapters that follow we will get to the bottom of what creates these conditions and what it is about our body, our brain and our behaviour that interacts to create a headache, and what we can possibly do about it. What is baked into our biology that makes us experience headaches (that we might not be able to change) and what is it about our environment (that we can change) that

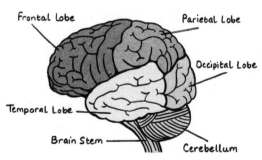

FIGURE 1 The Brain

means we often get them? This is where our most common solutions lie: either avoiding the headache altogether or heading it off before it takes over our lives. I warn you now: chocolate and sex feature prominently.

This book tells a story about what is going on in your head, your body and your life to cause headaches. If you are interested in migraine, by all means skip to Chapters 6 and 7. If tension headache is your nemesis, go to Chapter 4. Bear in mind though that the story builds as we go, introducing key characters that will have a role to play in later chapters. This is a story about you, and how all of you interacts to make you feel the way you do. If you are interested in the beautiful why of it all, start at the very beginning (it's a very good place to start!).

By the way, I never did find my glasses that morning. They turned up two days later in a shopping bag in the boot of my car only after my parents promised to re-mortgage the house and use the money to bribe St Anthony, the Patron Saint of Lost Things. I admit it would have been cheaper, but certainly not faster, to order a new pair.

2

Brain Freeze

TWELVE-YEAR-OLD MAYA KACZOROWSKI WAS OUT in the park one day with her parents, Janusz and Isabelle. It was a clear day in Hamilton, Ontario, and the family were discussing what Maya would tackle for her forthcoming science project. In common with many other 12-year-olds, Maya had no clue what to do. Her parents probed her interests. 'What do you like to do most in the world?' they asked. 'Well,' Maya said thoughtfully, 'I like eating ice cream.'

Janusz Kaczorowski was no stranger to the scientific process. Then an associate professor at McMaster University in Ontario, he worked in family medicine, publishing a wide range of studies about health through the life course and how general medicine should be practised. He was very familiar with randomised controlled trials and soon began talking to Maya about how she could set something up to investigate her passion. They decided to focus on ice cream headache. Janusz had told Maya that cold-stimulus headache (or 'ice cream headache') happens to about one in three people, but Maya was interested in what happened to this incidence when people ate their ice cream really fast (Maya used the technical term: 'gobbling'). Would an increase in ice cream headache experience in the gobbling group 'justify Mum's nagging' to slow down?

Maya and Janusz set about designing a study. First of all they had to create a pre-study questionnaire to see who had experienced ice cream headaches at some point in their lives, and a post-study questionnaire to see who had experienced one during the study. Janusz then helped Maya to figure out how to randomise her participants. In the end, they put a green or red dot on each pre-study questionnaire and flipped them over. If you found you had a red dot, you had to eat 100ml (3½ fl oz) of ice cream in less than five seconds. If you had a green dot, you could take your time and certainly not finish within 30 seconds. Maya ran the experiment by herself, explaining what needed to be done to her 145 willing participants, all students at Dalewood Middle School in Hamilton. She learned some experimental hacks along the way – scooping the ice cream was slower and less precise than cutting it from a block – and that things sometimes got messy in the gobbling group...

After six eating sessions, Maya had all the data she needed. She put it all into the computer for analysis and her dad taught her how to test for significant differences. It turned out that gobbling ice cream more than doubled a person's risk of developing a headache. These usually lasted less than 10 seconds yet were severe enough to cause 27 per cent of the gobbling group to clap their hands to their forehead in pain, as opposed to 13 per cent in the leisurely eating group. Interestingly, 79 per cent of her entire sample of schoolmates reported having experienced an ice cream headache before, which is higher than the figure random samples have shown up. This might be because children's experience of pain and their recognition of it is usually quite simple, and based on cause and effect: 'I ate the ice cream, it gave me a headache'. They also often eat it with great gusto. Another reason why there is a better recognition of ice cream headache in children is because in most cases they have few other pains to trouble them. How we recognise and remember pain is directly proportional to its effect on us, and this one makes itself known very forcefully and very fast.

Maya wrote up her study for the science fair. She didn't get awarded a prize but she's not bitter. She still got ice cream for her effort. Then her dad had the bright idea that they should write it up for the *British Medical Journal (BMJ)*. Every year, the *BMJ* publishes a Christmas edition featuring some papers that address popular conundrums in society. For example, a notable recent contribution concerned the possibility that vasodilation may have caused Rudolph's red nose, leading to a flurry of comments about the vascular system of reindeer noses in general. Maya's paper (which she wrote with some 'heavy edits from Dad') was entitled 'Ice Cream Evoked Headaches (ICE-H) study: randomised trial of accelerated versus cautious ice cream eating regimen'. It was peer reviewed for scientific rigour and published in 2002. By this point Maya was 13, making her the youngest author that I know of who has been published in the *BMJ*. That softened the blow of not winning the science fair!

The use (or abuse) of ice cream is not the only way you can demonstrate the cold-stimulus headache, but it is the most fun, which is why I endeavoured to replicate this experiment every year during one of the modules I was teaching at Durham University. I sometimes managed it, but more often than not I didn't.[1] One problem was that by the time we got to that part of the lecture, the ice cream was slightly melted and not as cold as it should be. The main issue, however, was that my participants were generally over 20 years of age and rather concerned about how they would look, which meant that getting them to gobble 100ml (3½ fl oz) of ice cream in five seconds was nigh on impossible. After a few years of this, I changed the experiment. Instead of ice cream, I brought juice boxes I had frozen in advance. By the time I needed them they were liquid again but still freezing cold. I also asked an assistant to squeeze all of the juice through a straw into their mouths either quickly or slowly. Boom, success! Groan city, but no chokers thankfully. The paperwork alone would have been a headache...

What is 'brain freeze'?

Lots of people call this the 'brain freeze' headache, but it is a bit of a misnomer. Your brain is not actually frozen. If it were, it simply wouldn't work and you wouldn't feel anything at all, or you might in fact be dead. (Although as a coroner friend of mine likes to say, you're not dead until you are warm, sober and dead. If your body is freezing cold, it slows down your metabolism to make your heartbeat much slower. If you are drunk, your heartbeat becomes faint, erratic and hard to hear, and your respiration slows down. Together, these two biological phenomena can make a body appear dead when it isn't.) While death by ice cream may be a wonderful way to go, it is pretty impossible to achieve unless maybe through obesity-related illness. Even more curious, the phenomenon is not restricted to ice cream or cold juice.

Surfer's skull

The phenomenon of 'brain freeze' is not restricted to those who gulp down ice cream or cold juice – it can happen to surfers and others who spend time in cold water, too. I often watch the surfers riding the waves near where I live, amazed that they can tolerate the chilly conditions. Curious about how they cope, on a cold March day in Saltburn-by-the-Sea, when the prevailing onshore wind had made conditions perfect, I intercepted a surfer called Mike as he came out of the waves and onto the beach. He wore a full wet suit with a neoprene hood on his head, boots on his feet and gloves on his hands; only his face was exposed. As a cold soul myself, I enquired as to his motivations for going out into the freezing North Sea in March. 'The buzz is amazing,' he said. Apparently the tides at that time of year, coupled with the wind direction, result in waves that are unrivalled anywhere in the world, and he has ridden them all. 'But, aren't you cold?' I asked. He gestured to his kit. 'No chance, not while I'm out there,' he said through chattering teeth (clearly dry land was the cold place), 'but the brain freeze is a killer.'

Even though Mike wasn't drinking from the North Sea, the very cold water was still getting into his mouth, where the temperature differential between the cold water and his nice warm neoprene-ensconced body could be as much as 30°C (86°F). Surfers tend to breathe through their mouths and so the water shoots in, in much the same way as juice through a straw, causing agonising pain in the temples. Mike even said the intense pain was the main reason he falls off his board, as his body temporarily stops functioning. Yet he and countless others carry on regardless – clearly, the buzz is worth the brain freeze!

Contrary to popular belief, the stabbing pain that you feel in your temples is not caused by sensitivity in your teeth but rather by overactivation of the sensory receptors in the roof of your mouth. Much of this has been described through painstaking investigation with crushed ice that Robert Smith did through the 1960s.[2] What Robert showed was that when ice touched the back of the roof of his mouth, otherwise known as the palate, pain came on around 20 seconds later as a stabbing, piercing sudden-onset sensation in the temple area above the eye closest to where the ice was located. Putting the ice anywhere else in his mouth didn't create the sensation. This is because the palate is the only part of the mouth that doesn't move, meaning it can give a really good indication, that's stable over time, of the temperature of the food or drink that happens to be in your mouth. This is important because substances that are too hot or too cold might cause damage to the soft tissue in your mouth, impairing your ability to taste properly. Our brain therefore needs to get some trustworthy indication of the temperature of substances in the mouth.

The gobbling that Maya investigated causes ice cream to be forced right to this sensitive zone at the back and top of the mouth, and the same is true of the cold juice that was squirted into the mouths of my students and the freezing seawater that enters surfers' mouths. Given the anatomy of the mouth and its connections to the brain, Robert concluded that the pathway involved is the sphenopalatine ganglion. This takes its name from the fact that it is located between the sphenoid bone ('spheno'-), which is behind your nose towards the front of your face, and the palate (-'palatine'); hence 'sphenopalatine'. A ganglion is a nerve bundle. This is where all of the cell bodies, or engines, of the nerves are bunched together, and it connects directly with something called the 'trigeminal pathway' (see below), which brings pain signals from the head and face to the brain. Activating this pathway, for instance by bringing something very cold into contact with it, makes your blood vessels dilate to restore the temperature and heal any damage the cold may have done, and this in turn tugs on the trigeminal receptors on the blood vessels as they get bigger. But why is the pain all the way up in our temple? Why is it not in our mouths?

To understand this we need to know something about 'referred pain', but let's start with thinking about the trigeminal nerve. This is a cranial nerve (a nerve that emerges from the brain) that controls all of the musculature in the face and head (including the smooth muscle in the blood vessel walls) and senses what is going on in the skin and musculature of the face, too. For example, it brings commands from the brain for things like the muscles of mastication (for biting and chewing) and expression (frowning and smiling) and takes sensory information back up to the brain, including touch and pain sensation. It's the largest of all the 12 cranial nerves and has three pathways in twinned directions either side of the face – hence its name (*tri*- 'three', *geminus* 'twinned') – and has dense pathways to the mouth and nose and also over most of the skull.

When the sphenopalatine ganglion is activated, the message is carried by the trigeminal nerve up to the brain, where it is lumped together with signals from other areas of the face. Your sensory system can't distinguish between these inputs and so we typically feel the pain in the temple area. Your body gets confused in other areas of your body, too. Much the same issue occurs when you feel pain in your heart from lack of oxygen, for example. Those signals are lumped in with the sensory information from your left arm and jaw, and so your brain feels the pain *as if it were coming from there.* Left arm and jaw pain are thus key symptoms of a heart attack.

There may, however, be a more direct reason why we feel pain in the temple region. In 2012, Jorge Serrador from Harvard Medical School asked participants to suck ice-cold water in through a straw and direct it to the back of their palate. They were asked to raise their hand when they felt the brain freeze come on. The researchers used ultrasound to track what was happening in the anterior cerebral artery – one of the main blood vessels bringing blood to the front of the head, which passes just behind the eyes. They saw a big increase in blood flow, caused by dilation of the blood vessels, before the participants raised their hand. Presumably it is this dilation that underlies the pain we experience. Once the anterior cerebral artery had returned to normal, participants indicated that they no longer felt pain.

So, we can say that brain freeze, or more specifically, the cold-stimulus headache, is caused by two things:

1 Overstimulation and referred pain from the palate. Since the response to pain in the body is always dilation, in order to bring all of the healing substances of the body to bear on the problem, the result is head pain.
2 A rush of warm blood to the head in order to keep everything functional. That rush of blood tugs on the trigeminal nerve receptors in the blood vessels themselves, also causing more pain, albeit through a whole other pathway.

This is why the cold-stimulus pain doesn't happen immediately – it takes a while for your brain to perceive what is happening in your blood vessels as pain. This pain lasts as long as it takes to regulate your blood flow. Usually by 10 (or maybe more) seconds after you have introduced the offending cold intruder to your buccal cavity (otherwise known as your mouth; 'shut your buccal cavity' stops any argument, period. You're welcome!) you will feel normal again. Thankfully, this two-pronged process is relatively brief. As we will see in the following chapters, some headaches are not so fleeting.

3

Sinus, Sensation and Snot

I F YOU EVER FEEL like you have been hit across the face with the back of a spade, there are two things to do. First of all, have a look around. Is there a possibility that you *have* actually been hit across the face with the back of a spade? If so, I'd run. If not, then the second thing you will have to do is consider the possibility that you are having a sinus episode.

A sinus episode encompasses both sinusitis, an inflammation of the lining of the sinuses, and the congestion that invariably follows. You have four groups of sinuses, which are air-filled cavities in the bones behind your face, with drainage ducts no bigger than the lead of a pencil. The biggest are in your cheekbones (called the maxillary sinuses) and those just above your eyebrows (the frontal sinuses). Ethmoid sinuses are found either side of your nasal cavity around the bridge of your nose and up in between your eyes. The last type, the sphenoid sinus, is behind the ethmoids. The sinuses all connect with your nose for the free exchange of air and mucus.

Light and strong facial bones

It often comes as a shock to think that the bones of your face are hollow, but it's not something to be worried about. The reason for it is so that your head is lighter, and the hollowness doesn't affect these bones' strength – just think of them as being a bit like the corrugated cardboard that protects goods that come through the mail.

And did you know that the strongest bone in your body is located in your skull? It's called the petrous temporal bone. Petrous comes from the Latin *petrosus*, which means 'stone-like' or 'hard', while 'temporal' indicates where it sits in the skull, i.e. covering your temporal lobe above your ear. Incredibly dense, rivalled only by the femur or thigh bone for strength, the petrous temporal bone carefully houses your inner ear, a beautiful spiral structure called the cochlea that converts sound waves into electrical signals your brain can understand as sound. The petrous bone is the last part of the skeleton to decompose, shows much better DNA preservation than other bones of the body, and so is a rich treasure trove for archaeologists. (It is also the only part of us that cannot be digested by sharks, as it happens; it's just too dense for their digestive system to cope with.)

The general symptoms of a sinus episode are varied. We feel it as a pressure in the face; tenderness to the touch, often escalating to facial pain radiating out from the sinuses; congestion and blockage of the nose; a bad taste in your mouth – accompanied by bad breath;

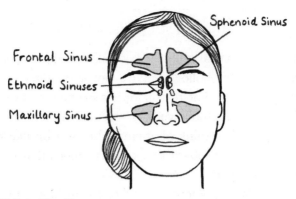

FIGURE 2 The Sinuses

an inability to smell properly, along with a productive cough that invariably keeps you awake; and of course the ubiquitous headache. We will talk about these in turn – but your biggest sign and orchestrator of all of these symptoms is simply snot. So, let's get to the core of that issue first.

Snot matters

I was always brought up to think that snot was a very rude word. My liberal parents didn't care, but my conservative school did and we were encouraged to use the 'proper' terms in language and not colloquial ones. (This was an inconsistent dictate, I discovered: the utterance of the word 'penis' was the quickest way to induce vertigo in a nun.) Besides, I dispute that the word snot is not proper. A Middle English word, it has been around since the late 14th century and means the perfectly descriptive 'nasal discharge or mucus'. The original root was *gesnot* for nasal mucus and this in turn came from an amalgamation of the German and Dutch variants of *snuttan, snotte,* and *snute,* all from the same base of snout, which makes sense. Old High German had *snuzza,* and still has the related *schneuzen* ('to blow one's nose'), and the Norwegians and the Danes use *snot* as a noun nowadays too. One word we did lose over the time since Old English was the verb *snite,* 'to wipe or pick one's nose'. I am rather gutted that this has gone out of modern parlance but will make it my mission to bring it back. Starting now.

When you feel the need to snite, it is because you have a build-up of mucus that is clogging up your sinuses and needs to be released. Mucus is released by epithelial cells, which cover the outer surface of the body as well as all of the internal organs and blood vessels and the inner surface of cavities such as the nose and the sinuses. Epithelial cells can look and act differently depending on where you find them, but in the sinuses they are shaped like columns and have tiny hairs, or cilia, on their outermost surface. These are the same kind of epithelia – called goblet cells – that you find in the upper respiratory tract, and have the power to secrete substances and move mucus around using their cilia. Although all of these goblet cells are securely attached to the surface of the bone surrounding it, if you look at them under a microscope, they appear to be layered or stratified, when they actually only consist of a single layer. The reason for this trick of the eye is because not all of the cells are of equal height, and the nucleus (or brain) of each cell, which is the most visible part of the cell under the microscope, can appear at different levels, helping the illusion that the cells are stacked in layers. So, we now know that the lining of the sinus cavity is made up of a single layer of ciliated pseudostratified columnar epithelial cells. The mucus these cells secrete acts like a protective balm; without it the underlying cells would dry and crack, which effectively flashes a big neon sign telling bugs where to attack since they can get straight in that chink in the armour.

Mucus protects in more ways than merely providing moisture, however. It is sticky and gooey, which is beneficial since particles get caught in it and don't go on to cause damage. Because the cilia of the goblet cells are constantly moving the respiratory mucus around (usually down the gastrointestinal tract but also out of your nose) these particulates don't get to hang around for long.

Mucus has other ways of defending us, too. It contains lysozymes – enzymes that make something happen. In this case, they break down the cell wall of any bacteria and burst the cell like a pin in a balloon. To top it all off, the presence of immunoglobulins or antibodies that latch onto and kill various incoming bugs means that much-maligned mucus has a premier role as our first line of antimicrobial defence.

We produce more than 1 litre (1¾ pints) of mucus a day from our nose and sinuses. This seems rather prolific, but you don't really notice it because most of it combines with saliva at the back of the mouth and is swallowed. However, when we have been exposed to a bug, or an irritant or allergen such as pollen, we produce even more mucus to defend ourselves, and the excess can trickle down the nose or run down the back of the nose to the throat – something that is called a post-nasal drip. The infection or allergy may also cause the lining of your sinuses to become inflamed, mainly due to the blood vessels to the nose and the sinus cavities swelling up. As horrendous as this sounds, this is the body's natural reaction to damage or infection.

First on the scene: histamine

Let's do an experiment. If you scratch your hand with a pen top right now, you will see a red line appear. This is caused by histamine, a powerful molecule that is stored in something called mast cells, which are tucked away under the skin's epithelial layer in this case. Histamine causes blood vessels to swell, making sure more blood is brought to the area of need (the bit of skin you've just damaged/irritated) and making the vessel wall leaky. This allows big white blood cells, which are the next line of defence in the immune system, to get to the area of possible infection. You see all of this as a pretty instantaneous red line on your hand.

In the nose and sinuses, the release of histamine makes the goblet cells produce even more mucus, which is now mixed with white blood cells called neutrophils. This can change the viscosity and the colour of the mucus you see when you blow your nose to relieve the inevitable congestion all of this causes, giving your snot the greenish colour it sometimes gets – because neutrophils have a green pigment in them. The histamine also acts directly on the sensory receptors in the nose, causing that itch and irritation that you feel. The congestion is mainly a vascular effect and the sensation of an itchy and scratchy nose is neurological. But how does all of this cause pain too?

The pain in your face

The pain that you feel when your sinuses are inflamed can vary, depending on which of your sinuses is most under attack. It is possible for all of your sinuses to be inflamed at once of course, but sometimes the mucus barrier that stops the epithelia in one of your sinuses from drying out and getting infected just isn't as efficient as the others, leading to a specific type of pain. For example, in addition to all of the other sinus symptoms, pain over the cheeks and just below the eyes accompanied by toothache and general headache indicates maxillary sinusitis, which makes sense because those sinuses are in the cheekbones. Frontal sinusitis, by contrast, localises your headache to your forehead. Given the position of the ethmoid sinuses, it isn't surprising that inflammation here leads to pain behind and between your eyes, and may also cause your eyes to water. This is the headache that most people describe as 'splitting', with the pain radiating to the forehead. Inflammation in the sphenoid sinuses that are behind the ethmoids leads to a more diffuse headache that can be felt in the front or the back of the head. This one is the most difficult to diagnose as the symptoms are more subtle and transient than those of the other sinuses. Trouble here can cause double vision and vision loss, and nasal discharge may or may not be present. The best way to diagnose problems in the sphenoid sinuses is to do an endoscopy, which involves sending a camera up the nose to look at the lining of this sinus to see if it is inflamed. This is always much more fun for the doctor than the patient, not least because the doctor gets to 'count your snots', or so I once heard an ear, nose and throat (ENT) doctor say to a patient.

Sinus pain vs migraine

There is some controversy about the headache that results from sinusitis, with many people who work in the field believing that 90 per cent of these may in fact be migraines, which we investigate in Chapter 6. The difficulty is that migraine can cause the same symptoms as those described above, including the generalised rhinitis – runny nose, pain around the eyes, etc. – which means that it can be hard to tell which came first. For both migraine and sinus headache, you might feel worse when bending over, due to the increased pressure in your sinuses. The symptoms of migraine, however, are much more severe than those you would expect with sinus issues, and the systemic (whole body) sickness of migraine is much more powerful than the general 'malaise' that results from sinusitis, mainly caused by digesting excess mucus from your post-nasal drip all day. Not the most nutritious of diets.

As we've already seen, the sensation of pain in your head is caused by the trigeminal nerve getting to work, and while the nerve carries sensory information from the facial region up to the brain, signals can also be sent *down* via motor nerves to the face and all of its structures. This can cause the confusion between a sinus headache and a migraine.

Let me explain further. With sinus headache, the nerve endings are activated by histamine and other inflammatory substances such as prostaglandins, and these signals are carried up to the brain and interpreted as pain. Just as in brain freeze headaches, pain can originate in the nasal area but be felt up in your forehead because all of the sensory nerves are lumped together in one tract and your brain finds it difficult to distinguish them. Conversely, with migraine, changes in activity in your brain cause the activation of the trigeminal pain receptors (or 'nociceptors'; from the Latin *nocere* for 'harm' and the English 'reception'), also causing dilation in the blood vessels below the epithelium, leading to the release of histamine and greater mucus generation and so on. So with migraine, instead of the problem originating in your nose and causing pain in your head, it is a problem in the brain causing effects in your nose.

Bless you!

The trigeminal nerve is critical to how snotty we feel, but it also makes you sneeze. It sends signals to your sneeze centre in the brainstem (yes, you have a sneeze centre), which organises signals to your head, activating the muscles required to open the nasal and oral cavities for a forceful exhalation of air to clear any obstructions or particles.

As we have already seen with referred pain, the trigeminal nerve can become somewhat confused. When it comes to sneezing, it can be triggered in several ways:

* The trigeminal nerve runs quite close to the optic nerve – the nerve running behind your eye – and sometimes, if you are suddenly exposed to a bright light, the abrupt activity of the optic nerve activates the trigeminal nerve. The brain interprets this as the presence of an irritant in your nose and so you sneeze. Aristotle suffered from this; he thought the heat of the sun on his nose was the problem. Sir Francis Bacon rather gleefully announced 2000 years later that Aristotle was wrong as he realised

that standing in the sun with your eyes closed made your nose warm but *didn't* cause you to sneeze. He was almost there in his interpretation of this, but not quite. He thought that the light would make his eyes water and that this moisture would seep into his nose and irritate it. The actual answer to the 'photic sneeze', as we now know it, has much more to do with fuzzy electrical activity in the brain than leaking liquid. It happens in about 35 per cent of people and is actually a genetic trait, like the ability to roll your tongue.

* Plucking your eyebrows also activates the sensory fibres of your trigeminal nerve, which are again misinterpreted as irritation to your nose, and can cause a fit of inappropriate sneezing.

* Some people are known to sneeze when they have a full stomach, a reaction that is not linked to the consumption of foods that actually make them sneeze by irritating the nose, such as mints or spices. Called 'snatiation' (a snappy blend of 'sneeze' and 'satiation') by geneticist Judith Hall, this response is genetic too, but its mechanism is less clear. It most probably has something to do with the trigeminal nerve travelling alongside nerves from the parasympathetic 'rest-and-digest' system.

* Unclear, too, is research showing the link between thinking about sex (particularly in teenagers) and sneezing, although again, crosstalk from the parasympathetic system is no doubt at play here. Next time somebody sneezes on the bus next to you, think about it. They might not just want to infiltrate you with their bugs…

A snotty slide

We get the same sinus reaction whether we are exposed to a bug or an irritant, but the reaction to an irritant should be more short-lived. I experienced this myself on a visit to a waterpark. It's not something I do very often – I may never do it again – but there is something fun about hurtling down a flume, even if somehow I managed to get stuck in one. I still don't know how that happened so we won't dwell on that part. It did occur to me, however, mid-hurtle, that there was an inordinate amount of water being forcefully introduced to my sinuses through my nose.

Picture the scene. I get very cold in water (a hangover from being a whitewater kayaker), and so I wear a lot.[1] However, I restricted myself that day to a swimsuit topped by a rash vest and water shorts. The wearing of all of these clothes that water doesn't naturally stick to meant that my downward motion through water on the flume effectively created an upwardly directed jet of water straight into my face. But it's just water, right? Wrong. Water is a great place in which nasty bacteria in particular can thrive and survive. Each new human body introduces germs into the water, and one person's natural germs are another person's pathogens... And then of course there are the effluents that come out of humans, such as mucus or urine. In response, most pools are treated with chlorine as a disinfectant to combat the pathogens, bacteria, viruses and fungi that are found in the water.[2] Chlorine combines with water to create hypochlorous acid, which attacks the bacterial cell wall, killing them by bursting them open.

So, not only are swimming pools and waterparks veritable Petri dishes, but they also contain chemicals to combat the bugs. All of this has the power to infect, in the case of bugs, or irritate, in the case of chlorine, your sinuses. The day after my waterpark experience, I therefore sounded like I had a heavy cold. My nose was blocked, there was congestion in my sinuses and I had a niggling headache in my forehead. This is hardly surprising, given the squirts of water up my nose that had flowed through the passages at the back of my mouth and then been swallowed. The same thing used to happen all the time when I was kayaking.

Here's an interesting aside, especially if you play or work in water. To combat the ingestion of possibly infected water from rivers, lakes and seas, particularly after heavy rainfall, thousands of kayakers and open water swimmers all over the world swear by copious swigs of Coca-Cola. Despite kayakers and swimmers feeling they have inoculated themselves against impending tummy trouble through the action of ingredients like phosphoric acid (rust remover – just try the rusty 2p left in a glass of cola overnight experiment if you don't believe me) found in the cola, there is no scientific evidence that this works in humans. The closest we have is a 2006 study by Eduardo Medina and colleagues from Sevilla, Spain who infected lettuce leaves with harmful bacteria and looked to see if Coca-Cola would kill the bugs. They also tested olive oil, vinegar, red and white wine, fruit juices, coffee and beer. The vinegar and the olive oil had the best anti-bacterial performance followed by red and white wine, which killed most strains after five minutes. All the remaining drinks had zero effect. The moral of this story is that kayakers and swimmers should chug olive oil or vinegar after a race or training session. Failing that, wine is a good option, a suggestion that made me very popular among my paddling friends.

In actual fact, though, our stomachs should in any case do a good job of neutralising swallowed respiratory bugs because our stomach acid is too harsh for them to survive in. The point is, there is no harm in swallowing mucus, or phlegm as it is also called. It's a good job, too, since we heard earlier in the chapter that we usually swallow about a litre of the stuff a day, and this is increased when your sinuses are producing more mucus. Each litre of mucus contains just over 200 calories, but I certainly wouldn't use it as a replacement for breakfast.

Right up my nose

What happens if we irritate our sinuses? If they are just irritated by the chlorine, for example, the inflammation in the sinuses should settle down after exposure because the immune system doesn't get involved. It's a good example of non-allergic sinusitis. However, the congestion caused by irritation can lead to an unwanted effect: everyday pathogens that would normally be trapped by the mucus and moved away before they have a chance to infect the epithelial cells get stuck because there is more mucus and it is moving less freely and not draining so well through the tiny (remember – lead-in-a-pencil-sized) ducts. Stuck bugs have more time to act and will cause infection, whether they came in with the irritant or were cold viruses that were sniffed up later. I was lucky: my congestion led to a mild headache and stuffiness for a day or two and then it resolved. No stuck bugs for me. And no, I haven't been back to the waterpark.

But why is it that something that is a minor irritant for one person causes an allergy in another? To answer this, we need to understand what an allergic reaction is: a heightened immune response to a substance. In the case of the sinuses, the most common allergen is pollen. You become allergic by changing your sensitivity to the allergen. Your body sees a seemingly innocuous substance like pollen to be an enormous threat and so raises antibodies in response to it. These immune markers then short-circuit your immune system, immediately indicating threat. That means that the next time you are exposed to the substance your body is ready and can swing into gear to fight this foe quickly and with everything you've got.

What makes your body decide that pollen is a bad thing in the first place, I hear you ask. Well, it seems to be mainly outside of your control, with genetics at play again. In 2012, Syed Hasan Arshad and his colleagues from the University of Southampton discovered that mothers seem to pass on their susceptibility to allergy to their daughters and fathers to their sons, meaning that allergies are carried on the sex chromosomes. There is still the chance that environment has a role to play here though, both while the baby is gestating in the uterus and in early life. Factors such as parental smoking, for example, or even experiencing a respiratory infection in their first six months can affect a child's risk of developing an allergy.

In addition to raising antibodies there is one other reaction mechanism your body can throw at pollen. Remember that epithelium layer in our sinuses and nasal passages? Well, beneath this layer is something called the sub-mucosa, where the histamine-containing mast cells live. In the case of people with sensitivities or allergies to triggers like pollen, these mast cells have migrated to sit *on top* of the epithelial layer and this is what makes people who suffer from hay fever extremely sensitive. The second that pollen is detected by the mast cells (and there is no barrier of the epithelium layer, remember)

BOOM, they dump out all of their histamine, causing the inflammation and the dilation of blood vessels and the leaking of white blood cells out into the mucus membrane.

It's a bug's life

The pathogens that cause sinusitis are generally viruses and bacteria. Bacteria will respond to antibiotics, but most viruses, including the cold virus, are very resistant to them and, unfortunately, most cases of sinus infection are caused by viruses.

The crafty cold virus

There are more than 200 viruses that can cause cold symptoms and sinusitis, the most common of which is rhinovirus, which only affects humans, chimps and gibbons (but not rhinos!). *Rhino* is a root Greek word for 'nose'. Rhinovirus is incredibly adept at infecting humans and has three main species types: A, B and C. Depending on the surface proteins these have, however, you can mix and match them into more than 160 different varieties. This makes it very hard to defend against them because your body raising antibodies to one type will not defend you against the other 159 types; you have to start all over again each time you encounter a new one. Ordinarily, if you are exposed to a bug you have already encountered and have antibodies for, your immune system swings effectively into gear, killing and carting off the bugs without you realising it is even happening.

The bugs can attack us directly causing a primary infection. We can make it easy for the bugs because viruses can easily get stuck – your body's gunky inflammatory response to something (like mine to swimming, for example). This then causes further congestion due to the immune response to the virus. But then other bugs can sneak in by stealth, like bacteria getting caught up in the congestion that is produced when the body is already busy fighting the primary infection. This is called a secondary infection.

Bacterial sinusitis is much more rare than viral infection of the sinuses, and is most common *after* a bout of viral infection. A typical culprit is *Streptococcus pneumonia*, more commonly named pneumococcus,[3] which can now helpfully be detected by a simple urine test. (It used to be that a nasal swab would be taken and the bugs on the swab would be cultured and grown in a Petri dish in a lab, which takes valuable time away from treatment.)

Haemophilus influenzae is an example of a Gram-negative bacteria (*see* box, p. 37) that attacks the sinuses. As you can tell from the name, it was (incorrectly) blamed for causing influenza; it was first described by German bacteriologist Richard Pfeiffer during an outbreak in 1892. However, by 1933 it was clear that the cause of 'flu is the Influenza virus, meaning that the original name of Pfeiffer's bacillus (*bacillus*: Latin for 'rod') seems more appropriate than *Haemophilus Influenzae*. Under the microscope, though, this bacterium looks like a hybrid of a spheres and rods, making it a 'coccobacillary', if we want to be really accurate.

Illuminating bacteria

When bacteria are isolated, you can look at them under a microscope. However, in order for them to show up, they need to be stained with various chemicals that cling to different parts of the cell, making them visible to us. In 1882, a Danish microbiologist called Hans Cristian Gram developed a way of doing just this, using a dye called crystal violet to cling to a component of the bacterial cell wall. Gram realised, though, that not all bacteria had enough of this component to survive the process of being got ready to be put on a slide for a microscope. These other bacteria did, however, react to a different stain called safranin, which turns them pink. In consequence, Gram realised there are two different types of bacteria, differentiated by their cell walls, and detectable by his stain. Cells that turn purple are Gram-positive and cells that turn pink are Gram-negative. When he published his work in 1884, he was quite downbeat about it, hoping that in another's hands it 'may turn out to be useful'. In fact, this turned out to be one of the understatements of that century; Gram staining is an absolute cornerstone of medical microbiology.

Both *S. pneumoniae* and *H. influenzae* live in the respiratory tract as part of our naturally borne bacteria or flora. (Yes, indeed, your tubes are a veritable botanical garden, with tiny living organisms dwelling in them.) These two, however, have a bitter rivalry over who gets to dominate in your airways. We know this because Christopher Pericone and his colleagues from the University of Pennsylvania introduced these bacteria to each other in a Petri dish in a really elegant set of experiments published in 2000. It turns out that *S. pneumoniae* destroys *H. influenzae* and a couple of other bacteria by releasing hydrogen peroxide, a fact that led the authors to reasonably conclude that this is how the presence of *S. pneumoniae* inhibits a number of other bugs also competing for resources in our upper airways. Then, in 2005, Elena Lysenko from the same Pennsylvanian team, led by Jeffrey Weiser, went a step further and introduced the bacteria to the real nose of a mouse. It turned out that strains of either *S. pneumoniae* or *H. influenzae* could colonise the nose quite efficiently if they were tested individually. However, when they were applied *together*, only *H. influenzae* survived after two weeks. It seems that *S. pneumoniae* started to attack *H. influenza* – just as Christopher Pericone and his team had seen on their Petri dish – but that this then triggered an immune response that specifically killed *S. pneumoniae*. It is therefore only the *combination* of the two species that sets off the immune system in this way. This is really important, because some of our treatments and certainly our vaccines are concerned with getting rid of one particular species of bug, when in fact we also have to be mindful of the secondary effects this can have, as a result of inadvertently changing the competition between existing bugs. There may be another, lurking, waiting to dominate when the competition is removed.

Although both of these types of bacteria cause a variety of symptoms, as the common cold virus does (but with more serious effects), *H. influenzae* is particularly likely to cause you a headache through sinus congestion. What's worse, Gram-negative bacteria like *H. influenzae* are harder to kill because it's really difficult to get anything through their cell wall, and also because various Gram-negative strains have acquired resistance to some antibiotics that used to work.

However, there is some light at the end of the tunnel. At the turn of the 21st century, researcher Terhi Tapiainen and her team from Oulu in Finland found that something as simple as xylitol, the sweetening component in your sugar-free gum that is also present in a small amount in your body, can stop both Gram-positive *S. pneumoniae* and Gram-negative *H. influenzae* from sticking to your mucus membranes. This built on work showing that the addition of xylitol in a Petri dish can inhibit the growth of both of these bugs. The dosage required to treat an infection would be quite high but could be administered in a syrup or chewing gum. Sometimes we use a sledgehammer to kill a gnat when all we need is a feather that was lying about anyway.

'snot fair

There are a number of other irritants that can affect our sinuses in a minor, albeit distasteful, way in comparison with allergic or infectious responses. We have all experienced changes in our mucus viscosity in extreme changes of temperature or when we enter a smoky environment, for instance, and perfume and paint fumes can cause similar responses. Other substances include alcohol or spicy foods.

Let's take the last example. I worked at Manchester University in the 1990s, and every week, my Greek friend Dimitri and my German friend Johannes and I would go a couple of miles south of the city to an area called Rusholme and in particular a street called the Wimslow Road. Here lies the Curry Mile, which boasts more than 70 restaurants dedicated to the cuisine of the Middle East and Southeast Asia. We went for the Indian curry. I was quite young and had never in my life experienced such tastes – the spicier the better for me. I loved it, but one thing was for sure – I needed to pack some tissues! This is because pickles, pepper and chillies all contain capsaicin and allyl isothiocyanate (which is also found in radishes and mustard) that protect the plant from being eaten by animals. Birds can eat as much as they like as they are not sensitive to it, so if your bird feeders are being raided by squirrels, just add chilli flakes. The birds won't mind, but the squirrels will go elsewhere. Both of these substances activate temperature sensors on your tongue, making you interpret them as hot, leading eventually to a numb tongue through overactivation of the sensory receptors. I enjoy radishes very much, but I learned the hard way not to eat a whole bag just before giving a lecture. My inability to control my tongue movements that day led to many a slip-up.

The most common effect of capsaicin is that it irritates the pain receptors of the nose, causing the rapid production of mucus. This is because such pain is interpreted as threat. It is no good having a beer with your curry to slake the heat, as you might think, because there isn't enough ethanol in it to grab the capsaicin molecules and they don't dissolve in water. Your best bet is milk; the casein found in milk loves fats and will hug the capsaicin molecules and rinse them out of your mouth. The traditional Indian yoghurt-based drink *lassi* is therefore ideal.

Drinks aside, all of these responses to spicy foods rarely lead to an episode of headache associated with sinusitis since the effects here are rhinorrhea, or runny nose, as opposed to congestion. Having said that, rhinorrhea can be used, however temporarily, to relieve stuffed-up sinuses, so it's worth cracking out the chillies if you have a blocked nose.

And then there's alcohol. Ever felt bunged up after a heavy night out? While some of you will swear that your sinuses clog up following a night on the beer, wine or champagne, there is little evidence in research literature to explain why this may be so. However, we can extrapolate from what we know is in alcohol and what we know triggers sinusitis and conclude that the typical culprit is histamine, the release of which is triggered by the ethanol in booze.

Why is this? Well, ethanol directly causes vasodilation in the blood vessels of the face, which tricks our brains into thinking we are under attack and causes the release of histamine, leading to the sensation of congestion both through the enlarged blood vessels taking up more space and the increased mucus release. But alcohol itself also contains histamine (as well as ethanol), which although metabolised by the stomach, may raise histamine levels in the blood over time. These histamines are also found in aged cheese, pickles, olives, avocados, sour cream and even bananas. Many of these foods have been implicated in dietary causes of migraine, too, further blurring the confidence that 'sinus headache' is unrelated to migraine if the headache presents on its own. In addition, the more alcohol you drink, the more dehydrated you get, making your mucus less runny and therefore harder for the cilia in your epithelial layer to move – leading to congestion as it all gets stuck up there rather than moving down into the post-nasal drip.

Sensitivities and sinus

Two other purported dietary demons for sinusitis are lactose, which is found in all dairy products, and gluten, found in wheat, barley and rye (bread and beer). However, there is a dearth of scientific medical evidence on this subject. What we do know is that some people have an allergic reaction to gluten – specifically one of its components, called gliadin – and this immune reaction causes inflammation in the small intestine, eventually leading to sufferers not being able to absorb nutrients from their food and resulting in the symptoms of Coeliac disease. But what about non-Coeliac consequences from gluten? Is it possible that the antibodies raised to gliadin or some other component of gluten can cause an inflammatory response in the sinuses?

One of the nasty consequences of raising antibodies to gluten is that they attack the intestinal lining, making a previously bumpy landscape, which is perfect for absorption, flat as a pancake. This is why Coeliac disease is called an autoimmune disease: it attacks your own tissues. The main class of antibodies that are raised are called Immunoglobulin A, or IgA for short. The thing is, IgA is also found in the mucous membranes of the respiratory passages and saliva and tears. The second immunoglobulin that is elevated in Coeliac disease is Immunoglobulin G (IgG), which is the antibody that is responsible for our immune reaction to pollen and pet dander (it is these tiny and microscopic flecks of skin that come off our furry and feathered friends that cause allergy, not the pet hair itself) and is found in copious amounts in all body fluids since it is our first line of defence against bacteria and viruses. So, is it possible that the elevated levels of IgA and IgG related to gluten (but which are not enough to cause Coeliac disease) can cause sinusitis? Thousands of people who have kept food diaries and tried restriction diets where they have systematically cut out gluten think so.

There is more peer-reviewed evidence in the case of lactose effects on sinusitis, with one paper related to this published in 2005; OK, not much more evidence than this one paper, but evidence nonetheless. Stephanie Matthews and colleagues from Cardiff University reported the case of a 53-year-old woman with lots of disorders and a 10-year history of asthma, eczema, sinus problems, muscle and joint pain and lack of concentration. She had been prescribed a number of pills, sprays and unctions and was on the waiting list for a knee replacement operation. Stephanie's team tested her for lactose intolerance, which involves ingesting 50g (2oz) lactose and analysing how much hydrogen gas is exhaled over the next three hours. If the value is more than 20 parts per million within three hours, it means you don't digest lactose well at all. Stephanie's patient's hydrogen level never reached this value and it was therefore declared that she was not lactose intolerant. The only problem with this was that the patient nevertheless suffered with a variety of symptoms after the ingestion of lactose, and these lasted for three days. So, the medical team decided to advise a lactose-free diet, just for a month, just to see.

One month later their patient was a new woman; the diarrhoea had cleared up, her skin was 'wonderful', her asthma and sinus problems disappeared and she was mentally less foggy and not worried she was getting dementia any more. Again, this resonates with many people around the world and brings into question what it is that we purport to be normal. While everything that we can measure medically has a 'normal' range, does that mean that you, as an individual, are represented within it? Our 53-year-old lactose-intolerant lady certainly wasn't and the proof was in the dairy-free pudding. The human body is as fascinating as much as it is a complex enigma. It's time we started treating people as individuals and not data points.

Your face's fault?

In contrast to these external causes of sinusitis, there are a variety of internal causes. The most common of these is nasal polyps. Originating most often in the ethmoid sinuses, they hang like teardrops from the mucosal lining. They are made of bits of debris, immune cells and connective tissue and are covered in the same ciliated pseudostratified epithelium that lines the cavity they live in. These soft and non-cancerous growths don't go away by themselves and can keep growing to block the sinus completely, in addition to having the capability to secrete mucus through their own goblet cells. They are caused by persistent sinus infections and allergic rhinitis, asthma and aspirin allergy[4] and are also prevalent in those who have cystic fibrosis.

The growth of our facial features up to and beyond adolescence can change the shape and indeed the existence of the sinuses. The ethmoid and maxillary sinuses (the ones around the bridge of the nose and the cheekbones) are there from birth but the sphenoid sinus behind your face only starts to grow at age seven and ends its spurt at the age of 15. The frontal sinuses only get filled with air from the age of four up to the age of 12, but they don't reach their final size and shape until we are 25; imagine the life you were leading in your early 20s when you thought you knew it all – and now you know that *part of your face hadn't even finished developing yet!* In addition to these structural changes, though, non-allergic sinusitis often happens during periods of hormonal imbalance, and particularly for females during puberty, menstruation and pregnancy, all the way from the second month of pregnancy until birth. Non-allergic sinusitis is also a symptom of an underactive thyroid gland, which leads to a slower metabolism. The mechanism by which hormone imbalance causes sinusitis is not really understood yet, beyond the idea that in response to such fluctuations the blood vessels of the nasal pathways enlarge, leading to an inflammatory response and a feeling of congestion. As if that person didn't have enough to deal with already.

The way it makes you feel

Those of you who have suffered from any of what we've covered in this chapter already know how pervasive a bout of sinusitis is; it might not be the most blinding headache you've ever had, but it is dull and it is always there, and in addition to the congestion, it means that extra energy is required just to go about your daily life. People who don't suffer from sinusitis sometimes have a lack of understanding about how it affects their friends, colleagues or families. However, now we have a questionnaire by which to measure the phenomenon (or 'phlegmomenon', as I like to call it). Questionnaires are tricky, because they ask you how you feel about certain things on a scale of usually 1 to 5. The answers are subjective of course, but filling one out does give a sense of how an individual is feeling over the period of time that the questionnaire is asking about; how their condition affects *them*. The same condition may affect another person less, or differently. This is the hard part: it doesn't reveal anything objective about how bad the sinusitis is;

only other tests like sending a camera up the nose could tell us that. It is therefore possible for somebody to score really highly on a questionnaire with the same physical presentation as someone who scores lower, showing that the former person doesn't cope as well as the latter. There may be many reasons for that. What the questionnaire *does* tell us is how the episode of sinusitis is affecting someone at a particular moment. Administered to enough people over time, a questionnaire's questions are tested for how reliable their answers are throughout a sample, and whether the answers are valid representations of their collective experience.

Jay Piccirillo, a head and neck surgeon and ENT doctor from Washington University School of Medicine in St Louis, Missouri, USA, and his team have since 1998 been developing the SNOT-22 as a questionnaire to test the physical and emotional impact of sinusitis. Don't you just love it when an acronym works out to describe what it is actually representing? In this case, it stands for Sino-Nasal Outcomes Test, and it features 22 questions relating to issues such as how bad your sneezing or runny nose is, through ear fullness and thick nasal discharge all the way to how fatigued you are and how it has affected your concentration, your productivity, your mood. These latter questions relate to quality of life; it is now clear that chronic sinus problems can severely affect you in ways that go beyond a ballooning of your weekly tissue budget.

The SNOT-22 in action

I gave the SNOT-22 questionnaire to a 52-year-old woman called Susan, who was teaching first aid to a bunch of us in my lab. She had been clearing her throat the whole time and sounded snotty and uncomfortable. During a break I asked if she had the dreaded lurgy (the cold that was doing the rounds). She said she'd had that about five weeks ago but this was just residual sinusitis – it always happened this way for her. What was very interesting to me was how it affected her daily life. Explaining that it was a bit of a drudge because she clearly wasn't 'sick enough' to take time off work, such a sub-threshold illness just had to be coped with, but it was both annoying and exhausting. She completed the SNOT-22 after the day's session and answered the questions relating to her experience over the last two weeks using a scale of 0 to 5, where 0 is no effect at all and 5 is as bad as could be. There is a maximal score of 110, given that there are 22 questions. Anything below 8 is non-existent, 8–20 denotes a mild problem, 21–50 is a moderate problem and anything above 50 is severe. Susan scored 61 – it's a severe problem – and got high (i.e. problematic) scores on all of the quality-of-life questions (except embarrassment; it has been bad for the last 15 years and so she is 'beyond that'). Interestingly, the worst quality-of-life issues that were flagged up related to sleep and fatigue. Poor sleep and not feeling rested can have huge effects on our ability to deal with life in general, never mind a chronic health issue. It can subjectively make everything worse and is a well-known contributor to depression, for example. The cause here for Susan was clearly the congestion, the post-nasal drip, the cough, the headache; the effect was a lack of good, restful sleep, and then that made the cause seem worse the longer this cycle went on.

I specifically asked Susan how she felt about the sinus headache. Her answer was that it was there all the time, usually a dullness or a heaviness. She had trained herself to ignore it but if ever she realised it wasn't there, she felt lighter and almost elated and found everything much easier to cope with. This is not unusual. Our brains can choose to ignore pain but our individual abilities to do this vary considerably. It is called pain gating. The simplest example of this is when we bang our leg on something and the first thing we do is rub it better. This works because the brain can't do two things at once – it can either receive the pain signal, or the feeling from your skin that something is touching it, and it is this latter 'somatosensation' that wins. This is a less obvious cure in the case of sinus headache as the source of pain is somewhat unreachable – you can't directly rub your sinuses. However, temporary relief *can* be gained by massaging between the eyes at the bridge of the nose and up into the eye socket where your ethmoid sinuses are, or even rubbing your forehead where your frontal sinuses are.

A higher-level example is the role of *attention* in pain. If you get to watch the television while you are sitting in the dentist's chair, I can predict two things. The first is that you are not with my dentist, and the second is that you will need less numbing agent because your brain doesn't feel pain as much because your attention is diverted. Susan is doing something similar, using her thinking brain, her sheer force of will, to ignore the headache caused by her severe sinusitis. Knowing that she is an ex-hockey player, I feel she has had practice building her pain tolerance...

I ask many of those I meet who suffer from sinusitis: are you sure your headache is a 'sinus' headache? Some ENT surgeons, like Nick Jones from Nottingham University Hospital, feel that 'sinus headache' in fact only happens in very specific cases, such as an infection in the sphenoid sinus, which is relatively rare. Is there the possibility that they are mixing it up with tension headache, as Nick thinks? Susan weighed up this question carefully. The tiredness and fatigue that sinusitis causes could make her more tense, leading to a tension headache, she thought, but her symptoms don't follow those of the classic tension headache, of which more in the next chapter. I hear this a lot. Some people are willing to say that their sinus issues cause head discomfort as opposed to pain; one young man said trying to make such a distinction was like splitting hairs and was entirely unhelpful. 'You know it was pain because when it is no longer there, it is bliss,' he told me.

Investigating sinusitis

What can be done for Susan and the countless others who suffer with sinusitis and all of its effects in both acute and chronic episodes? Given all of these causes of sinusitis, it is pretty clear that there is no one fix for this effect, so treatment must in part be related to its cause. As with all conditions, and particularly headaches in general, this is the key to their treatment. If it is not obvious to you then keep a diary and the cause should become apparent, allowing you to avoid your triggers. If not, it is time for an appointment with your ENT specialist, who can investigate for polyps or structural malformations for example, and whether or not surgery might be helpful.

In my conversations with Kate Blackmore, a specialised paediatric ENT surgeon, I learned about the diagnostic pathway in sinus problems. If a patient has a headache that is accompanied by other symptoms relating to the sinuses then it is easy enough to attribute the headache to the sinus problems. By the time a patient gets to her, they will probably have already been through a course of antibiotics, which will have made the patient feel better, indicating that it was indeed a sinus infection. Sometimes, a GP will have had a Computerized Tomography (CT) scan done too, 'to be helpful'. The problem is, these scans will only give you a snapshot in time, and one-third of all people at any one time will show some kind of massing of fluids. This doesn't necessarily signify anything; the rate at which our cilia move the mucus along means that in most cases this doesn't indicate any kind of underlying problem. Worse, these CT scans are basically three-dimensional X-rays, so repeated scans to check to see if the build-up is resolving are out of the question, unless you particularly want to glow from irradiation after a while.

Rather, Kate has become a detective, particularly in paediatrics with her younger patients, when they can't articulate what their discomfort or pain feels like. When I speak to people who work with children it always seems remarkable to me how much we have to experience pain in order to be able to talk about our experience of it. She told me this is why she loves ENT as a speciality; she gets to be a surgeon but there is also a fair amount of medicine involved, so she has to be interested in her patients as people. They hold the clues to their conditions. She needs to winkle out those nuggets and put them all together to make a diagnosis and then decide what the best route of treatment is for that individual. She asks lots of questions about the symptoms, onset and what the kid gets up to, for example. She will invariably stick a camera up her patient's nose to look out for anatomical issues or things that should not be there, such as inflammation, pus or polyps both in the nasal cavity and around the sinus ostia. It is the ostia (Latin for 'opening') in the bone that allows the air into the sinus cavities. She might also take some swabs to see if anything unusual grows in the lab.

Treating sinusitis

Sinusitis that is the result of allergy is easier to treat if it is caused by pet dander as opposed to pollen; ultimately, pets are easier to avoid. Kate says that she has seen a huge rise in allergy to dust mites (tiny relatives of spiders that feed on dust, which is made up mostly of flakes of dead skin we have shed) over her years of practice. The rise is still there even when you take into account better recognition of dust mites as an allergen in itself. There is still the prevailing view at the population level that this rise has happened because we are 'too clean', decreasing our exposure to dust mites so that our body sees them as the exception rather than the norm, mounting large immune responses when we are exposed to them. Some people I know, whom I won't name, see this as a great excuse not to dust. 'We don't want to disturb the dust mites, do we?' This makes as much sense as the five-second rule when you drop food on the floor. What? Is there a group of bugs with a stopwatch standing there saying, 'No, lads no, not yet... hang on ... 3, 2, 1 ... go for it!' I don't think so. But the point is that there *is* such a thing as being too clean.

Once you know what irritants trigger you then you should avoid them, if you can. However, for sinusitis following a cold and those things that you just can't see coming, there are a number of options. For example, if it's likely that you have a sinus infection (sinusitis that just doesn't shift for four weeks after the initial insult, such as a cold, for example), then antibiotics may be called for. Many diagnoses in general medicine happen by treatment. For example, if antibiotics clear up the symptoms in the patient and the pain and discomfort goes away, then it must have been a sinus infection. If not, there must be another cause.

Antibiotics and how they work

The most common antibiotic is penicillin, which was identified by Alexander Fleming in 1928. Penicillin and its relatives have something called a beta-lactam ring (oxygen molecules bound by carbon to hydrogen and nitrogen molecules) and these mimic a core component of the bacterial cell wall, helping them to bind to them and destroy their walls. Unfortunately, bacteria over the years have dealt with this threat by producing enzymes that can break down the beta-lactam ring before it can catch hold of the bacteria. In addition, penicillin has a much better action against Gram-positive bacteria than it does against Gram-negative bacteria as it finds it hard to attack the tougher cell wall of the latter.

People who are allergic to penicillin or for whom penicillin did not work may be prescribed a different kind of antibiotic, such as erythromycin, which has a slightly broader range than penicillin. It works by stopping proteins from being made inside the bacterial cell, preventing it from replicating. But again, these have limited success against tough-walled Gram-negative bacteria.

One antibiotic class that can attack Gram-negative and -positive bacteria is the tetracyclines, such as doxycycline, that were discovered in the 1940s, and act in a similar way to macrolides. However, these too have become less efficient due to bacterial adaptation.

Given the antibiotic resistance that many bacteria exhibit, a more targeted approach might be required. If the bacteria can be collected through a nasal swab and cultured and identified in the lab, the correct antibiotic treatment can be selected at the get-go. The problem is, this takes time – and often this is something that is in short supply, for a variety of reasons.

Doctors commonly say that people turn up at their surgeries in great discomfort and as a result they feel compelled to help them by prescribing something straight away. It's a human thing, they say. There is also the danger that due to the sinuses' proximity to the brain, bacteria trapped there can spread and infect the meninges or outer membrane of the brain (causing meningitis) or the tissues around the eyes. Therefore, if sinus problems cause you to experience severe headache, become confused or less alert and affect your vision, which could be dangerous, treatment is needed urgently. If you experience any of these symptoms, your nearest health professional should be your first call.

Surgical 'solutions'

Most of the interventions that ENTs will do for sinus problems involve prescribing medicines, as described, but if these don't work, then surgery is the next option. Historically, however, sinus surgery has been pretty brutal, focusing on widening the drainage ducts of the sinuses by drilling away the surrounding bone. This can be dangerous because there may be some collateral damage to other structures, such as the turbinates in the nose – bony structures that moisten the air as it comes up the nose. What's more, it's not usually appropriate for children because their faces aren't completely developed, and anyway they mostly respond to medical care. It is much more likely that ENT surgeons will operate on the children's adenoids (from the Greek *adēn* for 'gland') – little masses of tissue between the back of the nose and the throat that trap bacteria and viruses. Because of where they are, enlarged adenoids have the power to affect breathing and cause congestion, leading to a Darth Vader-type of respiration. Although enlarged adenoids might respond to a nasal steroidal spray, they ultimately may need to be taken out under anaesthetic.

What can *you* do?

We always like to think that the doctor is the last resort, so let's dwell instead on the things we can do for ourselves when avoiding the cause of sinusitis just hasn't worked.

Flush the bugs
The first thing to try is flushing out the sinuses at home with a sinus lavage, or nasal wash. It's very important that the solution you use is as clean as possible. You can buy sterile saline to use or make it at home according to your doctor's recipe, using boiled water, salt and bicarbonate of soda, with the resulting solution kept in the fridge. You can snuffle it up or you can use a teapot arrangement to squirt it up one nostril and out of the other, or you can buy a kit. This looks like an Olympic skill to me – I've broken my nose too many times to have this work personally – but it does have value; if you clear away stuck debris (which is useful by itself to feel less bunged up) before you take any inhaled medicine, there is more chance it will get to where it needs to be. You must be sure that your saline is as clean as possible though because you don't want to introduce more bugs where they are not wanted.

Menthol bungbusters

When I am feeling clogged up and have that 'hit across the face with a spade' feeling, I use a menthol stick, which merely requires you to insert the tube into your nostril and breathe deeply. These sticks are not to be confused with lip balm sticks (which treat sore, dry or chapped lips); even though they look the same shape, shoving a lip balm up your nose has less pleasant effects and if anybody catches you doing it, you will be teased unmercifully and, on balance, that is probably fair enough. But a menthol stick brings great and instant relief. How does it work? It stands to reason that the menthol is acting to dissolve the mucus plugs that are sitting at the bridge of my nose, doesn't it? Well, not exactly. This is one of those cases where reason does not predict reality.

Humans have been using this mint plant extract for hundreds of years in Asia, where it originated as a medicine for the treatment of respiratory diseases. In the Western world, however, it has only been used since the 19th century. These days it comes in many forms: vapo-rubs, sticks and sprays, lozenges, cough syrups ... the list goes on. What menthol actually does is act on the sensory receptors that detect coolness, which is why this is what we experience when we inhale it. So, despite menthol having *absolutely no effect* on airflow through your nose, you subjectively feel clearer. You don't *feel* bunged up any more.

What's happening here is that the menthol is influencing your perception of relief without affecting the congestion at all. It's selling you a dummy. Yet the perception that you *can* actually breathe decreases the inflammatory response from your brain, part of which was generated by you feeling that you couldn't breathe. Not being able to breathe through your nose is quite an emotional issue. It's stressful. Any stress will cause a stress response, the biggest effect of which is, yes, a rush of blood to the area. For this reason, feeling worried about not being able to breathe will make matters worse because it causes blood vessels in your head and sinuses to dilate, making the sinus ducts get even smaller. Menthol merely interferes with your perception of how bunged up you are, and in turn decreases this stress-related inflammatory response. The beauty of this is that even though you now know its secret, menthol *still* works. Our autonomic brain (the parts that keep us ticking in the background) functions without much interference from our conscious brain, and the cool receptors are all autonomic.

Menthol is only a relatively quick fix, and in the long term you will probably die of complications from Type 2 diabetes from all the sweetened menthol lozenges you are eating to control it long before you fix the sinus congestion. It is important to get on top of the congestion, though, because headache pain and dyspnoea (difficulty breathing) leads to fatigue and difficulty sleeping, leading to more fatigue. The body finds this stressful, making the inflammation worse, and distracting your immune system from fighting off other common bugs.

Make some space
What else can we turn to in our arsenal? Over-the-counter decongestants include pseudoephedrine (such as Sudafed) as an oral tablet (common in most cold and flu remedies), or oxymetazoline as a nasal spray. Both of these cause constriction in the blood vessel wall, creating more space to take in the air (unlike menthol, which just makes you feel like it has) by decreasing the space the blood vessel is taking

up. Another happy consequence is that by decreasing the blood flow to the area, the inflammatory agents aren't transported in at such a rapid rate, dampening the progressive bunged-upedness (this is my technical term).

Antihistamines
Also at our disposal are antihistamines. We saw earlier that histamine is a first line of defence in our immune system, a molecule that helps release white blood cells to fight infection out of the blood vessels by making them leakier and diverting more blood to the region that needs them by dilating the blood vessels. So, if you take an antihistamine, you cut off this inflammatory response at the knees.

There are two types of antihistamine. The one that was first developed will make you drowsy, as it crosses the blood–brain barrier and acts to decrease the histamine in your brain, whose role is to keep you alert. The other only acts to block the histamine receptors in the rest of the body and so decreases the inflammatory response there, but has no effect on your brain chemistry. The drowsy version is very handy when you want a good night's sleep to help you battle the effects of the bodily effort it takes to withstand the infection or allergy. The non-drowsy ones help with the symptoms during the day. Unfortunately, if you take antihistamine during pollen season, for example, you have to remember that you are decreasing your first line of defence to *all* threat. The most noticeable effect of this is that you will heal from skin scrapes and cuts more slowly than you normally would.

Rescue steroids
Man-made steroids act in the same way as our natural cortico-steroids, which are released by your adrenal

glands, which sit atop your kidneys. Made from cholesterol (yes, contrary to popular belief, it has its uses), cortisol is released in times of stress and has an important role in releasing energy into the body, reducing inflammation and constricting blood vessels as well as suppressing your immune system to focus on the stress at hand. Directing a dose of cortico-steroid straight to the area in which you have inflammation and a heightened immune response constricts the dilated blood vessels blocking your sinuses. What's more, over time the spray actually makes you less sensitive to what it is you are allergic to, be it pollen or pet dander. Most people just need short courses, however.

Kill the pain

Non-steroidal anti-inflammatories such as paracetamol or ibuprofen have more systemic effects, as they are taken orally. Ibuprofen, however, can cause breathing difficulties, particularly in those with asthma, as it causes airways to narrow in a condition known as bronchospasm, so for relief of a sinus headache, I would plump for paracetamol as the painkiller of choice.

Eating the problem away

If we think about inflammation as being central to the sinusitis experience, and working on the principle that a drug mimicking our body's own natural anti-inflammatory can be used to good effect, are there natural ways for us to increase the anti-inflammatory power of our own bodies? Remember, inflammation is a really important response to threat to the body, but sometimes, as in sinusitis – and indeed other conditions, such as arthritis – this becomes counterproductive.

Foods rich in anti-inflammatory properties should boost your ability to cope with inflammation. Omega 3 fatty acids, for example, have anti-inflammatory effects, and fish is a good source of this. Turmeric can also be used; there is evidence of such an application that can be traced to 4000 years ago in India, although there is more recent (250 BCE) evidence that it was used as a medicine in South Asia, mainly to treat poisoning. Today, there is a widespread use of turmeric, which contains curcumin as an anti-inflammatory, in alternative medicine. This use has been validated over the last 20 years; there have been a number of scientific papers that have defined the mechanism of the actions of this natural remedy both in a lab (*in vitro*) and in a living person (*in vivo*).

Earlier, I mentioned the role of capsaicin in making your nose run, hence relieving congestion. In contrast to menthol, we perceive this spice as heat. For a while, it looked like the application of capsaicin in the nose could be used in the same way as menthol, to trick the brain into thinking the air was moving more freely than it was. In 2015, Artur Gevorgyan and his team from Amsterdam reviewed the evidence and found that there was some value in trying it as a topical treatment, but the studies that have been done don't report objective measures such as air flow in the nose or levels of inflammation so can't be taken as gospel.

Bringing it all to a head

While it is pretty well accepted that allergic and non-allergic sinusitis could involve overly sensitive sensory pathways, we need more evidence to show how and how well these treatments actually work. This way, we can choose the right remedy for each person every time.

Despite a feeling in clinical and scientific fields that the sinus headache is a misnomer and possibly misdiagnosed when it is really a migraine or tension headache, the experience of the sinus sufferer indicates that it is a real and specific phenomenon for them. This is supported by the prevalence of other snitey symptoms in addition to the headache and the fact we know that what is going on in the sinuses of the face area is detected as pain in the head. If cross-diagnosis with a different headache is happening, it is much more likely that tension headache, rather than migraine, is the go-to alternative. We'll see why in the following chapters.

4

Stress and the Vicious Circle

I T'S FRIDAY. MY WEEK has been one of those where I had a plan. It was a good plan, a valid plan, an eminently deliverable plan. What I hadn't counted on was everything that was going to get in my way before I even got to the plan each day. Everything that got in the way was *urgent* and needed to be done *immediately* and I had to *drop everything* to do it. So, my plan to do all of the things I had to do anyway that were also *immediate* and *urgent* got pushed back. In addition, my heating at home packed up and that's been just another thing to get sorted out *urgently* and *immediately*. It's coming at me from all sides, and now, it's Friday and it hasn't stopped yet.

Here I sit with a pounding headache. It feels like I have an elastic band fitted tightly around my skull and there is a tonne weight sitting on the top of my head. I've done OK with getting everything done regardless of how much there was to do this week, but it has required late nights and working on my laptop in bed (it's freezing because of the heating problem). I know it's superhuman to get everything done and appear unflappable, but indeed it turns out that I am not from Krypton (Superman and Supergirl's home world); there is a cost and that cost is borne by me.

Part of this is emotional. Not only does my ever-growing to-do list and my ever-diminishing time stress me out, but I also don't really feel any satisfaction about managing it all. At least six people have asked me for something this week and it is in my personal nature to respond by the time they needed me to. *Urgently* and *immediately* of course. None of these people would have any idea of the requests of the other five, and so don't know that my efforts for them are Herculean in the face of all of the other pressures.[1] As a result, I don't even get the validatory shot of immense gratitude my emotional system feels it needs to compensate for the effort. And the cost is all mine. Is this sustainable? No. The graveyards are full of indispensable people.

We own our time. We must also own the consequences of our use of that time. We deal with stress constantly, so why is it that sometimes it gives us a headache? In this chapter, we are going to break down what it is about our emotional response to life that gives us a headache, and how that changes our behaviours to make matters worse. We will also think about how stress responses change our body posture and conversely how poor physical health can cause us to feel stressed.

Can you remember the first time you ever experienced a tension headache? They can be experienced at any age, but most people report the teenage years as the most common point of onset. I spoke to a group of seven-year-olds recently about their experience with headache in general. First, I asked them what a pain in their head felt like. Some looked at me blankly, which I took to mean that they had never experienced a headache, lucky tykes. Some described a 'thumping' when they got 'really hot' and didn't feel well at all. Having asked them why they didn't feel well, it turned out that these kids experienced a headache as part of a cold or other illness that caused a temperature spike. And then there were the kids who described tension headache as if they were reading from a medical textbook, which I am guessing they hadn't read at this stage in their intellectual development. Headache to them felt like somebody pressing down on their heads, and they put their hands up to their heads to show where the bottom of a hat should be. One child even went so far as to say, 'It's like if your hat is too tight.' Savvy kid. The children went on to describe a number of stressful situations they may have experienced, such as if there were loud noises or if they felt frightened or if they got into trouble or were falsely accused of something they didn't do ... the list went on.

I came away stunned by two things. The first was that in light of the plethora of causes I was given for their headaches they are ever well enough to go to school. The second is how amazing it is that a seven-year-old can attribute a pain in their head to an external event. It's easy to see how they can do this if they fall on their knee and it hurts, but they are describing how emotional events make them feel pain in a place they haven't bumped. This is phenomenal awareness for little people whose frontal lobes aren't yet fully wired up. If you are under 23 and reading this, don't get cocky; yours isn't fully functional either, which might explain some of the rubbish decisions you have made in the past. But that's an entirely different story.

The point is, even from this early age, we seem to attribute our headaches to emotional causes, and the biggest of these is stress. Stress isn't really an emotion per se, but it is our body's response to events our brains perceive as a threat to us. In my case this week, it was born out of having too much to do and not enough time to do it. This became emotionally tough because I wanted to do a good job in every task but felt pushed for time and the fear of not delivering made me tense. Or was it that in order to deal with what was on my plate my body went into fight-or-flight mode and it was this that my brain interpreted as tension? Let's break it down.

The body, the brain and the bear

The relationship between the mind and the body in emotion generation and perception has been a debate topic for thousands of years. If you see a bear running towards you down your local high street, you might think to yourself: 'That's unusual, what a lovely specimen'. Or, if you are not me, you might have a more 'Aaarrgh, I'm going to die' reaction. This is your brain's response to the bear, and your feeling of threat then kicks your autonomic nervous system into gear to release the neurochemicals (a chemical that affects the nervous system) and hormones required to give you the energy to get out of there pronto.

This theory of how we feel emotion was developed by Walter Cannon and Philip Bard in the 1920s. It stated that there is a physiological effect only after we have registered the emotion. This makes sense, although the prevailing view at the time was that of William James and Carl Lange in the 1880s. In contrast to Cannon and Bard, they thought that the sight of the bear would make you tremble, and your brain would interpret this trembling as fear.

Nowadays, we know that the brain and body work *together* to perceive our emotions. Given that the response your body has to a stressful scenario (releasing neurochemicals and hormones) is the same whether it is a good thing (accepting an award at the Oscars, for example) or a bad thing (seeing a bear on the high street), you need your brain to collect all the other information about what is going on around you in order to decide whether you are happy or frightened. What's more, it's worth knowing that our body *does* provide information to the brain about how worked up we should be. We know this because in addition to being paralysed physically, research has shown that people who have severe damage to their spinal cord feel less emotion about what is going on around them. The higher up the cut to the cord, the less sensory information they receive from around the body and so the less emotion they report that they feel.

It's a two-way street. The state of your body can make you feel stressed, and we'll come back to this when we talk about the role posture has in causing tension headache. Equally, your mind can cause your body to react with a stress response based on a previous bad experience.

The stress response is pretty typical in most of us, even if we all have different thresholds for when it kicks in. The most immediate response is the adrenaline rush to give us an immediate boost of energy to deal with a threat. The adrenaline kicks in so quickly that we might not even be consciously aware of our actions before we start to move, hence the historical confusion between James and Lange (body) and Cannon and Bard (brain). It is all controlled by the brain's perception through our sensory organs of what is going on. If you hear a screech and see a car careering towards you, your brain will quickly calculate whether it is on a trajectory to hit you and how long it will take to get to you. It will also work out what you have to do to get out of the way and set that in motion through the movement regions of your frontal lobe, causing you to jump out of the way of the car before you know what's even happening. We seriously are talking milliseconds here. In that fraction of a second, this information is also relayed to one of your emotion centres in your brain called the amygdala. Shaped like an almond (after which it is named), it is really active in our fear or threat response. Eventually, we will consciously perceive this as 'fear' but in the meantime, your hypothalamus will get kicked into gear by your amygdala.

I am not too proud to admit that the hypothalamus is my favourite part of the brain, full stop. It is like a command centre that sits behind all of the things that we subconsciously do. It controls a really fast neural pathway, the autonomic nervous system, which passes through the brainstem and down to the organs of the body. It also lords over our endocrine or hormone system, through its connections in the pituitary gland, and so it can influence when hormones are released. Both the autonomic nervous system and the endocrine system are important in the body's response to stressful situations.

The autonomic nervous system

The quickest response is through the autonomic nervous system, which has two complementary branches: the sympathetic 'fight-or-flight' system and the parasympathetic 'rest-and-digest' system. These two work together so that the body will be in the appropriate condition to deal with whatever is coming its way. When you are under threat, the sympathetic nervous system does many things, driven by the release of adrenaline from the adrenal glands that sit on the kidneys. This is a hormone that is also used as a neurotransmitter in the sympathetic nervous system, activating various organs to react. For instance, it causes dilation of your pupils by contracting the iris, or the coloured part of your eye, opening the aperture and allowing more light to hit the retina at the back of the eye. In much the same way as a camera, this means that you will get a much clearer and brighter picture than you did before. The pathway to your lungs also ensures that your bronchial passages are widened, allowing more air to come in so you breathe deeper and faster than usual. This influx of oxygen means your muscles and your brain will have the optimal levels right when they need to act. Glucose is released from your liver, the only fuel your brain can burn, and the quickest for your muscles to use. Your blood pressure increases as your arteries constrict, squirting blood to your organs quicker than usual; and coupled with an increase in heart rate you feel alert and ready to take on the world. Of course, you will also be sweating, have extreme piloerection and your mouth will be dry as a bone. Blame your sympathetic system – all that excitement sends your sweat glands into overdrive, causes the hairs on your body to stand proud (that's the piloerection) and inhibits salivary flow. I guess you can't have all the benefits AND be comfortable too.

The endocrine system

There is a secondary and more long-lasting stress response and again, it is mediated by the hypothalamus and the adrenal glands, but this time with a step through your pituitary gland. While the fight-or-flight response is controlled by your brain, the hypothalamic–pituitary–adrenal (HPA) axis response is *hormonal*, longer-lasting and has more consequences that result in tension headache. Your body is tightly controlled through feedback loops. If you are low in any of your hormones, a signal is sent to the hypothalamus to stimulate the pituitary gland to in turn stimulate the gland that produces the hormone you're low in to make more. When you have enough, the hypothalamus stops telling the pituitary to hassle the gland in question to produce more. The problem is that the HPA axis response works to keep the sympathetic nervous system response going and chronic low-level stress *keeps the HPA activated*. In essence, it means that your body is on heightened alert for a long period of time, and this can have many consequences for your health. Your blood vessels and arteries can get damaged through the fluctuations of adrenaline and this can have effects not only on your heart but also in your cerebrovascular system.

When you're in your stress loop the hypothalamus emits corticotropin-releasing hormone (CRH), which triggers the release of adrenocorticotropic hormone from the pituitary, which in turn causes the adrenal cortex to release cortisol. Cortisol activates systems in the body and is the main agent of our heightened alert state. It stimulates our body to replenish energy stores that are depleted during the stress and increases appetite so that we take on more nutrients to deal with the stress. However, most of the bears we are fighting or fleeing from are metaphorical so the intake of calories doesn't quite match up with the energy expended. This is one reason why a long-term effect of stress is weight gain, another reason being that cortisol prompts us to be ready with energy to run from the next bear round the corner too, and so squirrels away that extra calorific intake as fat.

Stress headaches and why they matter

So why does all this give you a headache? There are two ways in which the stress headache is born. The first is the effect that adrenaline has on our blood vessels. Adrenaline constricts peripheral blood flow – the blood flow to your extremities – which is why you go pale when you get a fright. It does this to redirect blood to more vital regions, such as your heart, your lungs, brain and the big muscle groups to help you get out of your situation by bringing more oxygenated blood to your heart, allowing it to beat faster, and your muscles, to help them work aerobically for as long as possible. As adrenaline fluctuates according to need, so does the response of the blood vessels. Over a long period of time, this can damage blood vessels, causing them to at best become less efficient and at worst causing them to break and leak blood. The latter can be catastrophic in the brain. Although we have known since Thomas Truelson's 2003 Copenhagen City Heart Study that self-reported high-stress activity and weekly stress was associated with fatal stroke, it wasn't clear that stress was an independent risk factor for stroke. Joanne Booth and colleagues from Glasgow Caledonian University reviewed the evidence in 2015 and found that how much stress people thought they were under was predictive of the incidence of stroke, but that the risk was higher in women. This tells us that there are more factors at play than simply adrenaline and blood vessels; the higher risk in women may be indicative of how women cope with stress through their physiology. One other mechanism is that we mount an immune response because we feel we are under attack. Indeed, in 2017, Ahmed Tawakol and his co-workers from Harvard Medical School linked the activity of the emotional regions of the brain to the overproduction of white blood cells, causing blockages and arterial inflammation, leading to higher incidence of stroke and cardiovascular incidents.

Our own *perceived* stress therefore causes an abnormal immune response, on top of the cortisol flowing around our system simultaneously ramping us up and trying to put out inflammatory fires. Your body is at war with your mind and when the body goes 'over the top' the immune response can even lead to complications that impede your recovery.

However, this is all a rather catastrophic view of what can happen with continued stress. Not all headaches result in stroke; this is an extreme, yet possible, outcome. We do have the power to avoid any of the factors that put us at risk of stroke. Tension headaches are possible side effects of stress and so should not be ignored. What's more, taken as isolated incidents, the headaches are unpleasant and scary in themselves and this adds to the general feeling of stress, which feeds into the circular problem.

A reminder: the pain in your head comes from the fluctuations in constriction and dilation of your blood vessels, which activates pain receptors. These signals are collated and carried by the trigeminal nerve, which you then perceive as pain. This tells you there is something wrong and that something in your brain is not working optimally; in this case, the something is the blood vessels' ability to bring blood containing vital oxygen, glucose and nutrients to your brain and leave again in an orderly fashion. However, there is another factor at play. Because of the constant stimulation of the sympathetic nervous system caused by the stressor, and also the pain signals from your blood vessels heightening your alert state, your muscles are more contracted than they ordinarily would be, constantly using energy and oxygen. Over a prolonged period, this leads to your muscles feeling harder than normal. It is not always easy for us to release this contraction simply by consciously sending a signal to our body with our mind. In fact, tense muscles can actually become a permanent feature in people who suffer from chronic tension headache.

Another bodily response to stress that has a role in how we experience tension headaches is the release of nitric oxide (NO). This is a gas found in the body that works as a neurotransmitter to relax the blood vessel walls, causing vasodilation and also inflammation. Patients who have angina will know that the GTN (glycerol trinitrate) spray, which delivers nitric oxide into the body, immediately widens the blood vessels that feed the heart muscle, causing instant relief from chest pain. It widens other blood vessels, too, which is why some people develop flash headaches as a result of its use. Indeed, nitric oxide has various actions that have been linked to different forms of headache. When we have a tension headache, nitric oxide that is released from our blood vessels seems to make us much more sensitive to pain in the tissue of the head and neck, including the signals from the tense musculature and the walls of the blood vessels. It even activates the trigeminal nerve directly. The vasodilatory effect of nitric oxide, meanwhile, has been linked to the mechanism of migraine, while the action of nitric oxide in the brainstem is correlated with cluster headache.

There doesn't seem to be anything good about the action of nitric oxide, does there? On the contrary: it acts with all of the other bodily systems to cause symptoms that tell us something is going wrong, and it also tries to fix it. One of the biggest roles nitric oxide has in helping us function normally is prompting recovery sleep after a period of no sleep, or sleep deprivation. Disturbed sleep is a huge stress for the body and may be severe in those who are under emotional pressure. And then there's the issue of fluctuating blood flow. Nitric oxide widens the blood vessels, which activates the pain receptors in the vessel wall. It also sets up an inflammatory response to deal with whatever is causing pain.

Remember, though, that at the same time cortisol is trying to reduce inflammation. The problem is, when you start to look at all of the systems that are trying to 'fix' whatever is not working properly in your body to cope with the effects of stress or pain you can often see a maelstrom of competing interests.

The painful cycle

As is becoming clear, cause and effect is cyclical when it comes to tension headaches. I'm still sitting here with my pounding headache and I am trying to reflect on which came first for me this week. I was mentally rushed, which I find stressful, and this has had a physical effect on me. I have sat for long periods of time, drinking endless coffees and not visiting the bathroom even when my bladder was screaming at me. It never occurred to me to stretch, who has the time? When I did need to go from place to place I have walked at full tilt, putting my unprepared muscles in a precarious position. In addition to my headache, I therefore ache all over and this hasn't helped my posture. I missed lunch most days and in order to wind down at the end of the day, I have sat hunched over my laptop in bed with a glass of wine (or two).

This time, my headache has been initially caused by a mental stress, a heightened alert born out of lack of time. But even without an emotional or mental cause, stress on the body can lead to tension headache all by itself. Posture, bad diet, dehydration, alcohol consumption, lack of sleep and the wrong kind of exercise all put the body and particularly the head, brain and neck region under stress, leading to tension headache. Together with mental stress, you have the perfect storm. I could feel smug about being thorough but really, I should know better than this; everything I did was wrong.

The physical causes of tension headache are well established. Jennifer Crampton, who has been a physiotherapist in Manchester for 20 years, says it can be related to many issues happening in the body; things like posture (when the usual muscles that keep us upright switch off, recruiting other muscles that are less suited to the job), alignment, pinching of nerves, overactivity of muscles, compensation of other muscles following injury and even the alignment of teeth and jaws. She is adept at finding trigger points – areas of hypersensitivity in the muscle when it is pressed – in her patients and these can often be in the neck area or the musculature supporting the head. When touched in this way, she can feel the muscle twitch and her patients report pain in their head, which is a kind of referred pain from the neck area. This all might be due to an injury or a repetitive strain; many of Jennifer's patients who are recovering from injury or operations that have affected their movement will present to her with tension headache and in this case she can take it as a symptom that something biomechanical may still need to be addressed. But Jennifer also raises an excellent point: what if postural changes are our body's way to relieve the tension in a damaged muscle and that is then causing the headache? In this way, the headache came first, leading to poor posture to try to correct for or mitigate the pain. Correcting posture without a good biomechanical view of what is happening elsewhere might therefore make the tension headache worse. I am now doubly convinced of the need for physiotherapists in this world.

Physical issues have knock-on effects on mental health and so should never be ignored or shrugged off. It is very common for Jennifer's patients to feel mentally stressed due to the bodily issues they are experiencing. The inflammatory response that is caused by a painful biomechanical problem that may or may not initially be making itself felt as a headache is interpreted in the brain as a negative emotion, usually as stress, thus increasing the problem and the incidence of tension headache. Emotional stress sets up an inflammatory response, too, in addition to the one the body is having in order to try to solve its physical problem.

Being hunched over a computer all day and then trying work in bed with really bad lighting won't have helped me. Because of the boiler packing up, my body was as stiff as a frozen fish stick anyway so there will have been a huge inflammatory response there, in addition to the inflammation I induced because of my many 'rushing around'-related injuries. I am also hitting that point in my life where my eye muscles don't work as well as they used to and so I suffer from eye strain a fair amount, another cause of tension headache. And to cap it all off, there is a building going up just outside my office and it takes a lot of effort to ignore the noise, which causes a stress response, too. Research shows that if there is noise of greater than 12 decibels when we are asleep, there is a marked physiological stress response; I was dealing with a much louder noise and I was fully conscious! *Ochón agus ochón* as we say in Ireland. Woe is me. Woe indeed, but a lot of this I could have alleviated myself.

What cost dehydration?

Drinking coffee and missing meals is no way to keep your body at peak optimal performance. Add to that a cheeky glass of wine of an evening and you are on the road to not providing the nutrients your body needs to cope with the stress response and repair damage, and you are also dehydrating yourself. I did drink constantly but caffeine and wine are both diuretics that make us urinate more (my poor bladder). And then, to add all of these insults to injury, I had a curry last night to 'do something nice for myself'. More stress on my kidneys trying to deal with all that salt and lovely spice. But what's that got to do with my headache?

Well, this might in fact be a dehydration headache, which occurs when we put our bodies through the kind of stress that I have this week, and often happens in combination with a tension headache, or is mistaken for one. As we saw in Chapter 1, your brain contains loads of water, which your kidneys draw upon in times of need. Thanks to all the water I lost by eating and drinking the wrong things, and the lack of replenishment, my brain volume literally shrank, pulling on the meninges and activating the pain receptors there. Not only that, but because my blood was more concentrated, there was less blood volume to carry nutrients and oxygen to my brain, however valiantly my vasodilatory system tried to redress the situation (leading to more pain from my blood vessels, of course). This made me feel foggy, wobbly and irritable. My heart was also racing because I had less blood, so my heart had to beat faster to get the same amount of blood circulating around my system. Little wonder then that my sympathetic nervous system interpreted all of this as a threat.

This is the vicious circle of the stress response and it is hard to know whether it is the body or the mind that is more rancorous. The answer is, we can't think about the brain as being separate to the body either when we are thinking about what causes headaches or thinking about how to deal with them.

Want some cheese with that whine?

We make bad choices when we are under emotional stress, often and especially when it comes to food. We eat poorly, which when tied up with the cortisol released by the hypothalamic–pituitary–adrenal (HPA) axis response means we gain weight. We drink more alcohol because we think it will help us to relax; we are not really wrong in that view – alcohol is classified as an anti-anxiety agent and sedative hypnotic after all – but there are some other things we should take into consideration when we use it in this way. A couple of drinks will activate the inhibitory neurons in your brain by mimicking a neurotransmitter called gamma amino butyric acid (GABA) and this gives you a more relaxed experience, which can lead to euphoria, or withdrawal, or even violence, depending on the setting. If you have more than a couple of drinks then the receptors for glutamate, one of the main excitatory neurotransmitters in your brain, are blocked, making you feel much less anxious and even sedated because there is even less activity in your brain than normal. Increasing inhibition (through GABA) and decreasing excitation (by blocking glutamate) both feed into how alcohol makes us feel. We often become disinhibited when under the influence of alcohol and that's because the part of your brain that controls judgement, the frontal cortex, becomes selectively turned off, while the subcortical structures are spared. This means that the part of the brain that is responsible for our more primitive instincts, such as desire, is still active. These regions also control the dopamine reward system, which also stimulates the production of serotonin (the happy hormone) and endorphins, our natural painkillers. Our actions feel good and all is right with the world. And yet, we don't have our frontal lobe working to tell us right from wrong. And we might get lost, a lot. And we might not remember anything. It explains why when we have been drinking, we tend to make bad decisions, like to eat from the kebab van parked outside of the bar, or to go home with someone we wouldn't ordinarily consider. This is the neurobiology of beer goggles.

Coming down off a busy day with a glass of wine is one of the great advantages of being a grown-up, but it doesn't take long before one glass of wine doesn't work to make us feel as good as it used to. Our tolerance changes, we create more endorphin-binding sites, so it takes *another* glass to feel as good as we used to. So now, we not only have more dehydration to deal with, but we also have a chemical conflict in our brain. Once we stop drinking and externally controlling the neurotransmitter levels, overnight our brain realises that now it is just not excited enough. In consequence, it works to bring GABA (the inhibitor) levels down and boosts glutamate (the excitor). This results in an unnatural environment, which we interpret as anxiety, that can last for a couple of days. David Nutt from Imperial College London coined the term 'hangxiety'. That glass of wine you thought would help you wind down has actually maybe made things worse.

On top of all of this, alcohol is a diuretic that overcomes the usual body clock suppression of urine release overnight. Four hours after slipping into a blissful and restorative sleep, you wake up needing a wee. But by now you feel bad about yourself and even more anxious about what you have to do the next day because this is when the GABA/glutamate imbalance kicks in as well. Great, not only are you awake, but you also have to get up and visit the toilet, *and* you are stressing out. The sympathetic nervous system kicks in to try and be helpful and now that's the ball game.

I'll admit I haven't slept very well this week. I do wake up early when I have a lot on, but this week I've been waking earlier than usual and had no luck getting back to sleep. Nitric oxide must be flooding my system, trying to be helpful and get me some rest, but of course it is messing with my blood vessels, too. My immune system will be releasing inflammatory agents and I am tired, and not prioritising well, taking longer to do things than usual. Add to this all of the other things that I have done wrong this week, and the result is that I have a banging headache by Friday. As a kick in the teeth, the so-called weekend tension headache (which should actually be renamed the downtime headache to cover all work patterns), happens as your body and your brain is readjusting to its baseline levels and repairing and restoring function. Part of this is the inevitable inflammatory response and vasodilation in the cerebrovascular system, leading to the cruelty of a headache in your free time.

Arresting the stress

Some physical causes of tension headache are easily dealt with. A new chair leading to better posture and a better prescription for your eyes may just change your life! However, conditions such as arthritis of the cervical area of the spine in the neck are harder to tackle because your immune system has turned on the connective tissue in the joints between the bones of the spine, degrading the cartilage cushion and causing inflammation and pain.

Mental causes that set off the cascade of physical events that are interpreted as stress by your brain are less well defined. We don't often enough link our physical well-being to our perceived stress levels and vice versa. Tension headache sufferers I speak to tell me that they only realise they have been under 'too much strain' when they get a blinding headache. Joining the dots for them is always instructive. You were worried about x, or you have too much on. You dealt with everything, but you ate badly, slept badly and you were not hydrating or exercising properly. Your brain interprets these signals as threat, increasing the stress response.

Where in this process do you think you could have avoided a headache? Most of the people I talk to in the course of my work say 'by remembering to eat right or drink more water', or 'by exercising' – in effect, optimising their ability to deal with the stress that seems inevitable to them. To a degree, this is true. Our jobs require more and more from us in less and less time. Not all of us enjoy our jobs, which means we don't get to counteract the stress with little shots of dopamine and serotonin during the day. Many of us have parenting or caring responsibilities in addition to our paid work, making us feel torn, displaced and guilty.

We have oxytocin to thank for this one. A fine hormone that promotes bonding not just between lovers but parents and children, it can cause a feeling of unease when you are away from your paramour or offspring. We learn to deal with it over time – I think even the least cynical of us would agree that it doesn't last long in new relationships – but it is much longer lasting when it comes to our children.

Chill, baby

Over the years that I've taught a course on headache, pain and drugs, I've asked my students why they didn't just relax a bit about what was causing them stress. I was careful with my language here – I learned a long time ago that it is unwise to tell anybody in a tizz to 'calm down'. Although there is no scientific literature on the consequence of this, my own experience has shown that it leads to a motor response that somewhat resembles a right jab. Nobody *chooses* anxiety, so telling people to chill out once it has happened is pointless. But what about trying to lessen the fight-or-flight, or HPA, response to stressful situations where a big physical effort is not required? How might we do this? *This* is the key to prevention.

The trick here is to reassert the conscious brain's control over unconscious processes. This is as hard as it sounds, and requires self-awareness and practice. But master it and it will give you the best of both worlds: you will have the cognitive alertness when you really need it, and adrenaline and cortisol will be released to give you a boost. Even better, that control will mean that not every little thing will cause a big stress response in the body, with effects that result in headache. You really do get to choose what you worry about, and know what it is you cannot help but worry about.

Clinical psychologists call this 'resilience' – the ability to cope with a crisis or to return to pre-crisis status quickly. I would actually go half a step backwards and ask if what you are experiencing is a crisis at all. There are the obvious ones we cannot help but raise a stress response to, such as illness of a loved one, bereavement, worry about the whereabouts of a child late home from school, climate change – we need our physiological response to deal with these crises – but some other examples I hear about are no big deal compared to these, and often dependent on the stage of life people are at. Certainly, my involvement with education has made it very clear to me that emotional development is just as important as, if not linked with, intellectual development. And so I have developed a five-point plan:

Resilience 101:

1 Don't sweat the small stuff.
2 If you are not in control of the situation, don't worry about it. Worrying won't change it.
3 Just think about the next step and not the myriad consequences that may be a consequence of all of its consequences.
4 Prioritise, starting with family first.
5 When I look back on this in a week's time, will I wonder what all the fuss was about? Take the long view.

All of these will help you measure how much of a stress response you should mount, and with practice it becomes pretty automatic, leaving you calmer, with a bit more space than you used to have when you jumped into situations feet first. The five-point plan works for most things, but even recognising when you worry about things outside of your control (such as the health of loved ones) can help you put your stress response into proportion through the other behaviours of the plan.

The medication route

There are medical ways to do this. Beta-blockers decrease the activity of the sympathetic nervous system and stop your body from mounting a stress response, which makes you feel calmer.[2] Anti-anxiety medication that changes the levels of neurotransmitters in your brain is also widely used in treatment. Drugs that increase the amount of GABA, or decrease the amount of glutamate action in your brain will result in you feeling calmer, but you will need to take more to get the same effect as you adapt.

These medications may help you get a handle on how to deal with the emotional causes of your stress, but they won't make them go away. The lasting effect comes through the changes that you make to your behaviours to allow you to sustain a chemical balance in your brain naturally. Johann Hari speaks about this eloquently in his book *Lost Connections*. Everything from dealing with past trauma, through building resilient behaviours to social interaction can be used as ways to rebalance your brain in the long term. Learning how to deal with and respond to the *emotional causes* of stress is the key. And we have to do this through behaviour. Drugs can help us be more receptive to this learning and get us out of an emotional hole but they are not a long-term solution on their own.

Meditate on this

A less medical approach but one that is no less fascinating to a neuroscientist is meditation. Techniques that focus on breathing are there to slow you down metabolically. A reminder: if the sympathetic nervous system is in gear, we will breathe faster than usual. Consciously slowing down breathing lessens the perception of threat by the brain, and decreasing the inflammatory response, particularly to the brain, where dilation causes pain.

Meditation can change the balance of your neurotransmitters but, given time, will also change how your brain is wired up. I've mentioned before that the frontal cortex contains the part of your brain that helps you make decisions and rationalise what is happening. It also houses the bit that works out how everything that is happening relates to you. As part of the emotional, or limbic, system, the insula, which lives deep inside our brains, is very important in our emotional responses, self-awareness and regulation of the body's state. The amygdala, which we have already met, is also critical in our first reaction to situations. Ordinarily, the medial (middle) frontal regions communicate extensively with the insula and amygdala because it is important for us to see how stimuli, be they internal like heart rate or external like an approaching bear or deadline, are going to affect us in particular.

Sara Lazar from Harvard Medical School has scanned long-term meditators and has found that what meditation does is strengthen the control that the lateral (areas to the side) frontal regions have over the medial region. The lateral frontal regions give us the context of what is happening. Over time meditation enables you to look at what is going on inside and outside of your body more objectively. In the same way that your frontal lobe helps you bite your tongue when your emotions really want you to let rip with a few curse words, in this instance, the lateral frontal lobe takes the sting out of your emotional response, preventing the sympathetic nervous system and HPA from escalating the situation. Even better, by strengthening the pathway between the different regions involved, our empathy for others and our social connections are enhanced. Sara also saw lesser amygdala activity (the area that becomes active in response to threat) in consistent meditators. This field of research is about 20 years old now and is moving on to look at the difference between various meditative techniques such as yoga versus mantra-based methods, and to find out how long the effects last for. One thing is for sure: 50-year-old meditators have the same grey matter volume as 25-year-olds, showing that there is a neuroprotective element to it. Once we know the mechanism of this, we will understand why.

Training your body

Other techniques focus on breaking a stress response through a physical action that you have associated with something that makes you feel happy instantly – installing a feeling of calm instead of anxiety. Psychologists call it 'classical conditioning', most famously demonstrated by Ivan Pavlov and his dogs. Every time Pavlov presented food to his dogs he would ring a bell. After some training, every time he rang a bell his dogs salivated as they expected food. The previously neutral stimulus, the bell ringing, became a conditioned stimulus for salivation. Salivating in response to a bell wouldn't be so good if you found yourself in a stressful situation – and so you make your own association. By training yourself to associate a feeling of happiness with a physical action such as touching your nose or pulling your ear lobe, you can trigger these feelings to mitigate stress in the future. Every time you feel happy, tug on your ear lobe. After some weeks of doing this, if you feel anxious or stressed, tug on your ear lobe again. You should now be releasing those neurotransmitters that are unleashed when you are happy and this dopamine and serotonin gives you the capacity to deal with what's in front of you more calmly.

Breaking bad – what to do when you have a tension headache

Once you have the tension headache, though, we have to break its resultant vicious circle somehow. There are various ways of doing this. For instance, relaxing the body through massage, heat treatment or stretching (which arrests the contraction in our muscles) will decrease the pain signals from the musculature and so the resultant vasodilation in the head.

Most of us, of course, instead reach for the painkillers. Ibuprofen, paracetamol and aspirin are the main over-the-counter medications for tension headaches. All act to reduce inflammation, with ibuprofen having the strongest action. However, as we have already found, it can cause stomach irritation and wheeziness in asthma sufferers. Aspirin can also be harsh on the stomach lining, with paracetamol (known as acetaminophen in the US) the best tolerated by the gastrointestinal tract. Most of these will also come delivered in a pill containing caffeine, which works as a vasoconstrictor (constricts the blood vessels) and also helps the drug's movement through the gastrointestinal tract. However, taking regular tablets with water followed by a coffee on their own would suffice – just remember to drink more water afterwards to counteract the dehydration the coffee will cause!

Wired to the moon?

Caffeine withdrawal headaches are also a thing, particularly in heavy coffee drinkers. I had a student who once piped up in class that if she didn't have coffee within half an hour of getting up, she got a headache. I asked how many coffees she would have in the day. The answer was a whopping 13 mugs! Her headache was being caused by the fact that her blood vessels had gotten used to being constricted all the time. When that external constriction was released, her blood vessels dilated, sending warning pain signals. This was too much to bear for my student which was why she drank so many coffees. Such withdrawal effects are a huge component in addiction – and she freely admitted her addiction to caffeine.

Paracetamol: pain and empathy killer

There is something really interesting about paracetamol, and this could also apply to other over-the-counter painkillers. Dominik Mischowski and his team from Ohio University have shown that people who have taken paracetamol are *less empathetic to other people's pain*. This isn't trivial; empathy is a big part of why we behave the way we do towards others and so paracetamol's ability to manipulate this might be seen as a social side effect as opposed to the physical side effects clinical trials usually monitor. Dominik's view is that because a decrease in perception of pain (through the action of paracetamol) is linked to a decrease in acknowledging the pain of others, there must be a shared mechanism between the two in the brain and that this is a basis for empathy. We already know there is a sensory component of pain (what does it 'feel' like?) involving sensory regions of the parietal lobe, but also the frontal regions we've just talked about, and the limbic system, too. But there is also another pathway that is much more subcortical, involving a region known as the 'zona incerta', which is very important in how we experience pain. What may be a tickle for me may be excruciating for you. Activity in the zona incerta is modulated by many factors, such as your levels of circulating endorphins (natural painkillers) but also your experience, your upbringing, your educational status, your social position, your diet and your relationships. In a further study, Dominik found that participants who had just taken paracetamol are less sensitive to the pleasure they would usually gain from happy stories (called positive empathy). So perhaps feeling happiness shares a mechanism with being able to detect other's emotional states.

There is a lot more to do to confirm these findings and also we have to bear in mind that in this experiment the paracetamol was being taken by people who were not feeling pain to begin with – and so its effects may be different if they were. It is also interesting that despite paracetamol being developed by an American chemist, Harmon Northrop Morse, in 1878, and first used clinically by the German Joseph von Mering in 1893, it remains a bit of a mystery. *We are still not completely sure how it produces its effects.* We know that its anti-inflammatory action happens at the level of injury, blocking the release of prostaglandin, which begins to heal damaged tissue causing the inflammatory effect. By stopping this effect you effectively halt the pain signals from being generated there. But certainly in some people, paracetamol acts in the central nervous system, too, boosting the serotonin pathway from the brain to the body, otherwise known as the descending pathway, which blocks the ascending pain signals in the spinal cord – the ones coming up from the body to the brain. We know this to be true because if you block the serotonin receptors, you can stop paracetamol from being as effective a painkiller. This is useful to understand – especially because anti-emetic (anti-nausea) drugs are packed full of these serotonin receptor blockers, but are frequently given together with paracetamol post-operatively. This means that one of the ways in which paracetamol works is cut off. Go figure. This illustrates why understanding mechanisms is so important.

Paracetamol also encourages the activity of your natural endorphins, making them hang around in your synaptic clefts (the gaps between your neurons) for longer. This may be dependent on your natural levels of endorphins but it would seem to explain the feeling of relaxation and even euphoria that some paracetamol users report, even outside of its painkilling effects.

One last mechanism worth mentioning is that paracetamol would seem to block our old friend nitric oxide, too. Nitric oxide synthase inhibitors (or, put another way, drugs that stop nitric oxide from being produced) have been suggested as a treatment for tension headaches for 20 years. Development has been slow, though, no doubt due to the many effects that nitric oxide has in our body, leading to lots of side effects if we block it medically. And of course as it turns out, paracetamol may already be blocking nitric oxide anyway!

Immersion therapy

If all else fails, settle down and watch a movie. Movies are medicine. Seriously. By taking your mind off the pain and diverting your attention not just from your aching head but also from what caused it to ache in the first place, you will feel better in no time. Watch something funny; laughing gives you a quick hit of serotonin that will make you happier and block those pain signals. It also helps to drink water, watch your posture (unless you are being hugged; never turn down safe oxytocin, that's my motto) and wear your glasses. Oh, and eat a couple of squares of chocolate – that boosts serotonin too. It all helps and it's what I am off to do right now.

5

The Cacophony of Cluster Headache

Y FIRST EXPERIENCE OF cluster headache
was when I was 25 and working at Oxford
University. I was just going back to the lab after
lunch and as the lift door closed, I caught sight of a student
I would later find out was called Rachel, sitting hunched
on a chair at a table, and literally banging her head against
the wall with the 'Encapsulated Asbestos' sign on it. I hit
the button to open the doors again and approached her
cautiously. There is always that part of you that thinks if
somebody is upset they probably just wish to be left alone,
but there was something about the involuntary nature of
her movements that alerted me. Besides, if she didn't want
me to be there, she'd tell me to go away and this was the
only course of action I could live with.

I sat down next to her and at this point her forehead was
on the table; I couldn't see her face as her hair was all over
the place. The gentle touch of my hand on her shoulder only
elicited a groan, as if I had made things worse. Eventually,
she raised her head and began a rocking motion; she was
clearly very upset. It was when I looked more closely that
I realised Rachel had a droopy left eye, that was watery
and very bloodshot, and she was extremely flushed and her
nose was all stuffed up. She also appeared panicked when I
looked into her eyes. I jumped to the conclusion that she

had been attacked and at least punched in the face, or had fallen down the stairs. None of this was true. 'I have a headache, it feels like it is going to explode. It's the worst I've ever had. Nothing helps,' she whispered, clutching the left side of her skull as if trying to keep its contents in. Welcome to the world of cluster headache.

What is cluster headache?

There are several common descriptors of cluster headache, which was relatively ill-defined and unknown back when I encountered Rachel in the lab (we are talking 20 years ago).[1] One of my favourite of its many monikers is *Erythroprosopalgia of Bing*. It sounds very sci-fi, but I am not sure Paul Robert Bing, the titular German/ Swiss neurologist active in the early 1900s, would be very impressed with my categorisation. It really just means redness (erythro-) of the face (prosopo-) with pain (-algia). Then, in 1926, Willfred Harris, a neurologist based in London, called it migrainous neuralgia, further confusing it with the migraine experience. This was followed by Horton's Cephalalgia, or the catchier Horton's Headache after Bayard Taylor Horton, who described its pathogenesis (development of a disease) in 1939. I find it hard to believe that anybody would want something so unpleasant to be named after them, but whatever twists your biscuit, I suppose.[2]

The most anatomically descriptive moniker for cluster headache is sphenopalatine (a group of nerve cells that are connected to the trigeminal nerve) neuralgia, but that doesn't do it for me either because it is too narrow in its focus. By 1953, however, Edward Charles Kunkle had coined the term 'cluster headache', since they tend to 'cluster' together over time, both within a day and at certain times of the year, and this is the term I use. Eventually, this led to the formation of the Cluster Club[3] in 1974, led by Norwegian neurologist Ottar Sjaasted and of which academic and clinical researchers were members. It was very clear that interest in headaches had been exploding since 1960 with societies and associations springing up on both sides of the Atlantic. Ottar would later go on to navigate a political storm to unite global headache researchers under the International Headache Society in 1983.

Over the years, our understanding of cluster headaches has changed radically. Many factors are now considered when it comes to working out what causes them. Back in Horton's day in the 1930s and 1940s, histamine was identified as a culprit, reflected by the seasonal nature of the onset of a cluster of headaches (they tend to be more common in the spring) and the specific symptoms they display. But over the years, genetic abnormalities, activation of the autonomic nervous system, hypothalamic function and other factors have all been brought into the explanatory mix. There are some lifestyle factors, too, the main offender being smoking, but also alcohol. So, first of all, let's think about how the cluster headache presents itself and how people experience them, so that we can decide what effect each cause has and what we can do about it.

What cluster headache looks like

Headaches have to have particular symptoms to be considered as belonging within the 'cluster' class. Rachel, the girl I met in Oxford, was a pretty classic presentation, except for the fact that cluster headache is four times more common in men than women. You have to have reddening and watering of the eye, a runny or blocked nostril, a drooping or swollen eyelid, constriction of the pupil, flushing and facial sweating. In addition, the patient will be restless and often be rocking or pacing up and down. They will describe the pain over one of their eyes and towards their temple as excruciating and as if somebody is either trying to push their eye in or out of their socket. This only happens on one side or the other but has been known to switch sides within an attack. Of course, given its name, when, how and how often the headache presents is also a key distinguisher from migraine. Attacks have to happen between one every other day and up to eight a day, and there have to be at least five attacks with the symptoms described above at any stage before a diagnosis can be made.

These symptoms have been defined as cluster headache since 1998, when the International Classification of Headache Disorders (ICHD-I) first recognised it as a disorder in its own right. Since then there have been two ICHDs, with the most recent ICHD-III in 2018 recognising two variants according to whether it is episodic (at least two cluster periods lasting from seven days to one year, separated by a pain-free period of greater than one month) or chronic (which occurs without a remission period, or when pain-free periods last less than a month and this has gone on for at least a year) in nature. But what is happening in the body to cause all of these effects?

The causes of cluster headache

The first clue lies in our genes, for it is by the action of these that proteins are created – the building blocks not just of how we look but also our bodily functions. The reason we suspect genetics is because 5–10 per cent of cluster headache patients have a family history of cluster headache. It is likely, though, that there are many genes that have a part to play.

A quick bit of biology background: we have 46 chromosomes in each of our cells (23 pairs), but only 23 single, unpaired chromosomes in each of our 'gametes' – the ovum or egg cell for females and the spermatozoa for males. When the male and female gametes fuse, we get a merging of these chromosomes into 23 pairs (so 46 chromosomes in total) and this is how we end up with half of our chromosomes coming from our male parent and half from our female parent. Twenty-two pairs of chromosomes are autosomal (non-sex). The other pair is the sex chromosomes; you have two chromosomes that look like Xs if you are genetically female and one shaped like an X and one like a Y if you are a genetically male. And sometimes, as in the case of cluster headache, genetic abnormalities can be passed on with all the other traits (*see* pp. 157–161 in Chapter 7 for more about traits).

Now, some traits are dominant, which means that you only need to have the gene from one parent in order for it to be expressed in the resultant child. If a trait is recessive, though, you need that gene to be passed on by *both* parents in order for the child to develop the trait.

However, although it's true that the traits that are coded by the 100,000 genes on each chromosome make us who we are, there are other factors at play, too. The biggest factor is known as epigenetics, or factors that affect whether genes are turned on or off without affecting the DNA sequence. This is why cloning rarely results in genetically identical organisms that look *exactly* the same, completely nixing the plot of many B-movies – a plot device that always makes me throw my popcorn at the screen. The prenatal and postnatal environment and even how parents interact with their offspring can change how proteins are made through gene expression without changing the DNA structure of the chromosome. So we, and our actions, are created every day by an intimate interaction between our genes and our environment. Patrick Bateson, a zoologist from Cambridge, has a lovely way of putting this. We all start our lives with the capacity to develop in any number of ways; we have the ability to play any number of developmental tunes. Patrick calls it the 'developmental jukebox'. Crucially, though, it is our environment that picks out the tune. This doesn't mean that genetics don't have a part to play, they do –it is your genes that determine what kind of developmental tunes you have stored in your jukebox from which the environment can select – but epigenetics takes care of the rest.

So, we mustn't have tunnel vision about genetic causes. Yes, an abnormality may indicate a propensity to a particular trait or disorder, but we also need to think about under what circumstances that trait is expressed and if there is anything we can do through our environment or behaviour to stop that. In the case of cluster headache, the gene that has the most evidence for involvement is the one that creates a receptor for orexin, also known as hypocretin. This means that orexin has more of an opportunity to influence what is going on in the brain. Catchily called the HCRTR2, it is an autosomal dominant gene (meaning it is not on the sex chromosomes and you only need it to be passed from one parent), and it is also polymorphic, meaning there are different variants of what this gene looks like. Some of these variants may alter how the receptor that is made acts, by changing how receptive it is or what the receptor will accept. The science is ill-defined as yet and not constricted to HCRTR2, but let's follow this particular rabbit down its hole a little further.

The orexin gene has a role that is mainly played out in the hypothalamus, where it helps to regulate feeding behaviours but also lots of other things, such as sleep–wake regulation, mating and maternal behaviour.[4] Orexin is released in higher concentrations after a period of food deprivation but it also responds to the taste incentives of a particular food. Let's say you are in a restaurant and have had a lovely meal and then the waiter brings you the dessert menu. Given that waiting staff work so hard, it would be rude not to look, of course. And then you spot the chocolate fudge cake served with Madagascan vanilla ice cream. Orexin has the power to override any satiety indicators that are reaching your hypothalamus, allowing you to 'find room' (presumably in the separate compartment in your stomach reserved for dessert) even though you are completely stuffed.

Orexin also has a major role in the reward system for substances other than food, such as alcohol, nicotine and drugs like cocaine. Jessica Barson from Drexel University in Philadelphia and Sarah Leibowitz from the Rockefeller University in New York believe that orexin production is kicked into gear by exposure to such substances in early life, and so the environment has a role. Perhaps, then, it is no surprise that the incidence of smoking in those with cluster headache is about 90 per cent in males and 70 per cent in females, which is much higher than the rest of the population. Even exposure to second-hand smoke as a child has been linked to cluster headache prevalence. But instead of thinking of nicotine as a *cause* of cluster headache, it may merely be correlative due to the action of a more sensitive HCRTR2 receptor for orexin. This idea seems to be validated by smokers themselves. Anna Ferrari and colleagues from the University of Modena, Italy, admit that even though smokers seem to have a more severe experience of cluster headache, stopping smoking does not prevent it from happening.

And, as it turns out, those who suffer from cluster headache and those who treat them believe that alcohol is a trigger for cluster headaches. The early research indicated that not only were you more likely to be a heavy smoker but also a 'hard drinker' too. But instead of alcohol being a trigger, one way of looking at it is that through the abnormal action of the orexin gene, it is easier for these individuals to become addicted to, say, nicotine or alcohol, but neither of these substances is actually driving the bus to cluster county – orexin is.

Smoking and alcohol can have negative effects on any headache, though, and so it is possible that they may induce even more negative effects in cluster headache. Nicotine, the psychoactive drug contained in cigarettes and the more modern vapes,[5] acts to constrict blood vessels in the cerebrovascular system. Blood pressure increases, meaning the heart has to pump harder. With long-term use, carbon monoxide levels build up in the blood to exceed those of people who live in the most industrialised cities in the world. Both of these factors have the effect of starving the brain of optimal amounts of oxygen. This can lead to migraine, as we will see in the next chapter, but for all other types of headache, the rebound vasodilation triggers the pain effect, just like we saw in sinus and tension headache.

The light link

The way our body and brain reacts to light is another clue. Our natural circadian rhythm would actually dictate a

26-hour day, but this happens only if we live in a bunker with no natural light at all, and who wants that? Light acts via the non-image forming cells of the retina, which signals the suprachiasmatic nucleus (SCN) that lives in the hypothalamus (the centre of our hormonal system) to conform to a 24-hour cycle, roughly related to the amount of day and night that exists on earth. The presence, or absence, of light therefore constrains this cycle and so is termed a '*Zeitgeber*' German for 'time' (*Zeit*) 'giver' (geber). The SCN isn't just a clock, it's also a pacemaker for many other biological rhythms happening in the body. One of the biggest of these is our sleep/wake cycle. When light levels decrease, serotonin is converted into melatonin in the pineal gland and is released into the bloodstream. This acts on the inhibitory mechanisms in the brain, promoting sleep. In high-light-level conditions, serotonin is *not* converted into melatonin and so wakefulness continues.

In the winter, when there is less light, particularly at higher latitudes, there is the tendency for more melatonin to be released. This is an evolutionary trigger – winter means hibernation and conservation of resources. In humans, however, this can be counterproductive to modern life, and the greater production of melatonin and therefore lesser concentration of serotonin (the happy hormone) can lead to Seasonal Affective Disorder (SAD). You could therefore reasonably assume that the darker the season the higher the incidence of SAD, but this is not always so. While the prevalence of SAD in Finland is 9.5 per cent, there are few reports of SAD in Iceland, which is at the same latitude. Dietary differences may explain this phenomenon; Icelandics eat much more fish than the Finns and so their diet is richer in vitamin D. Vitamin D regulates our absorption of calcium, which is critical in how well our neurons communicate both with each other and with our muscles, and it seems to have a protective effect against SAD. So, a better diet can fix part of the problem, although we also need to increase the amount of light entering our eyes. If you are not in a position to visit sunnier climes twice a year then exposing your eyes to a light that is a tenth as bright as the sun for 15 minutes a day in the morning using a light box will help kick your SCN into gear.

In cluster headache sufferers, fluctuating light levels over the year might explain the periodicity of clusters that sufferers experience as they may find it difficult to regulate their hormones in response to light. Such rhythmicity also explains why cluster headache often occurs while sufferers are asleep. We have different phases of sleep, ranging from Stage 1 to 4, during which our brain activity gets slower and slower. In between we have periods when our brain shows the same activity as if it were awake, and this is called rapid eye movement sleep or REM. All the other stages are non-REM. Towards the end of the night our sleep becomes dominated by REM sleep, which is why we can often find ourselves dreaming as we wake up. We do dream in non-REM sleep, too, but they tend to be more methodical and even nightmarish. With REM sleep, the frontal lobe isn't active at all, and so nothing makes much sense; it's also harder to remember the dreams. The onset of cluster headache is often reported to occur during REM sleep when the brain is more wakeful, and towards the end of the sleep cycle when circadian hormones released to wake the body up are at their peak.

There is another curiosity here: if we tie in the fact that four times the number of males experience cluster headaches than females, you might think that this is related to some kind of sex-linking of genetics, that the trait is mostly passed down to male offspring. However, there is little evidence for this. A more tantalising link is how sex hormones interact with the SCN, particularly testosterone, which is released in much greater concentrations in males than females. Even though the male and female SCN has the same volume, it is more elongated in females than in males, where it is more spherical. The interaction of sex hormones and the activity of the SCN and the knock-on effect on our behaviour is most apparent in teenagers of both sexes – puberty being a veritable hormonal hurricane. It resets the body clock of your average teenager forward by about two hours, which means that their biological day starts at 9am rather than the more usual 7am for adults.[6]

Post-puberty, females release hormones cyclically while males release theirs in a more constant way. Bayard Horton back in the 1930s and 1940s and others since have identified that there is a decrease in testosterone release in males who suffer from cluster headaches. Testosterone concentration is ultimately controlled by the hypothalamus by an area called the preoptic nucleus, which happens to be twice the size in males as it is in females. This is an area that is active in sexual behaviour but also body temperature regulation when we are ill. (I once got into bother by joining these dots and speculating that this may be why many males of our species experience 'man flu', but I digress.) A malfunctioning hypothalamus might explain lower secretions of testosterone but also how that then affects the SCN, as testosterone has the ability to organise and change the function of this central biological clock. A lack of testosterone may disrupt our normal rhythms, causing non-typical bodily changes for the time of day/year we find ourselves in – explaining the clustering of the headache.

You might therefore think that the answer is to administer additional testosterone to bring levels more in line with 'normal', but this doesn't seem to have an effect on cluster headache prevalence. However, in this small study involving seven patients in 1993, Maria Nicolodi from Florence University, Italy, and colleagues showed that the top-up testosterone did increase patient sexual excitement when compared with that of patients in the control group who didn't have any additional testosterone, so there are hints here that it is involved in some part of the pathway. (So perhaps you can just self-medicate through sex; more on that later.) Of course, the level of testosterone depletion is key, and as with many drugs, so is the timing of the administration in relation to the body clock; there is no one-size-fits-all solution here. Work needs to be done to tie all of these threads together.

The histamine alliteration

Another clue comes from histamine, the molecule that we discussed with respect to allergy and sinus headache. Since the time of Bayard Horton's research back in 1939 histamine has been thought to have a role in cluster headache. The increased temperature on the painful side of the forehead and the coincidence of flushing led him to implicate histamine as a vasodilator, and to use the term histaminic cephalalgia (from the Latin *cephalo-* ('head') and *algia* ('pain')) when describing it. Somehow, Horton's Headache is more catchy, and Horton's Histaminic Headache has a nice ring to it even if the alliterative police are probably now rolling their eyes. Whatever the name, Horton realised that his patients may have an extreme sensitivity to histamine. In support of this conclusion, he noticed that many also suffered from stomach ulcers, a condition in which histamine has a big role, as ulcers are inflammatory responses to the *Helicobacter pylori* germ.[7]

So, histamine is a by-product of the stomach ulcer, but what Horton had realised was that raised histamine was also coincident with headache. Just to be sure, he also injected histamine just below the skin in his patients and caused many of the symptoms of cluster headache in some of them. What's more, he had also noticed in his male patients that gastric acid secretion was higher, which is controlled ultimately by the hypothalamus, and testosterone release was depressed, also controlled by the hypothalamus, particularly during an attack.

We also know that histamine controls wakefulness through the hypothalamus working in concert with orexin/hypocretin and the serotonin–melatonin balance described earlier. What controls the action of all of this? The answer: light, entering the eye and being processed by non-image forming retinal ganglion cells reaching the suprachiasmatic nucleus (SCN) of the hypothalamus. And so we have come full circle.

Further still, Marcello Fanciullacci from Florence University noticed a difference in pupillary responses in sufferers back in 1979, with the pupil on the headache side in his cluster headache cohort being smaller than the other pupil. Pupillary response is an automatic reaction controlled by the autonomic nervous system and its malfunction can be seen in other aspects of the cluster headache symptom suite; activation of the parasympathetic system causes the teary eye and the runny or blocked nose, and deactivation of the sympathetic nervous system causes the droopy eye and the smaller pupil. And what controls the autonomic nervous system? The hypothalamus! While we have been occupied with investigating different aspects of the problem, we have been pretty blind to the entire picture. Such is the way of science.

In conclusion, each of these aspects, in particular the vasodilation that results in activation of the trigeminal pain pathways and the influence that each of these hypothalamic functions (histamine, autonomic involvement, serotonin imbalance, orexin sensitivity) has can be persistent and colossal in magnitude.

The hypothalamus hypothesis

So, what is the evidence of hypothalamic dysfunction being a cause of cluster headache (as opposed to the sub-components above)? What do we already know? The hypothalamus *can* affect things that are happening on the same part of the brain (usually, everything is crossed over with the right side of your brain controlling the left and vice versa). In addition, we know that the hypothalamus has a fast-track connection with the trigeminal pathways responsible for the pain and also that the hypothalamus has a big role to play in dampening down pain signals – if it is working properly. In 1998, Arne May and colleagues from the Institute of Neuroscience at University College London induced cluster headache in people who suffered episodic cluster headache using nitroglycerine (remember, nitric oxide is a powerful inducer of headache through the rapid vasodilation it causes) and put them in a Positron Emission Tomography (PET) scanner, which tracks the flow of radioactive water that has been injected into the patient prior to the scan. They compared the activity seen in this group with that of a group of cluster headache sufferers who were not currently in pain. They could see an increase in functional activity in the hypothalamus during pain periods but also structural changes in the hypothalamus, particularly in the bit where the SCN lives.

Others have debunked this idea, however. More modern imaging like functional Magnetic Resonance Imaging (fMRI) does not rely on the injection of radioactive water but instead works by analysing what water molecules in our bodies do when a radio wave is applied, having first pointed them all in the same direction using a magnetic field. What results is a picture that is much clearer than one we could achieve with PET. Steffan Naegel and his colleagues from Essen, Germany, didn't see any difference in size of the hypothalamus in cluster headache sufferers in 2014, but *did* see differences in other areas of the brain, such as the temporal lobe, hippocampus (important for memory), insular cortex (part of our emotion system) and the cerebellum (important in eye movements and balance) – all of which can have roles in the behaviour of cluster headache sufferers, such as rocking, restlessness and irritability.

What is critical about this much bigger study, which involved patients at different stages in the disease and also within and outside of pain bouts, is the finding that brain structure is dynamic and reactive to the environment in which we find ourselves. Many parts of our brain will react to pain strengthening the response of some areas over others to allow us to try to control this abnormal activity that is causing pain in our body. It is this dynamic that has made it hard to define a causal link with the hypothalamus. We need to know more about how these different areas of the brain talk to each other, why and how they get so chummy. But if there is a way to control the symptoms that are tugging on all of these different networks throughout the brain, we need to go to the puppet master, and all accusatory fingers right now still point to the hypothalamus.

You might have been wondering what happened to Rachel, the girl last seen banging her head off the wall. Well, I managed to take her up one floor to my office and sit her down with something cold against her face. Thankfully, she was registered with a GP practice (you would be stunned by how many students who are living away from home don't do this). I looked up their number and gave them a call, describing her symptoms and asking if she should go to the hospital or to the doctor's surgery. They told me to send her to them. In the end, I had to put her in a taxi for two reasons. The first was that I rode a motorbike at the time, and even though she had recovered somewhat, I really didn't think she could cling on behind me properly, so I couldn't take her that way. The second was that I had a participant coming to see me in the lab so that I could run an experiment on him. Given that I was planning to send magnetic pulses into his head, I didn't want to muck him around too much by cancelling. Besides, by then Rachel was feeling a bit better; the droopiness in her eye had gone away, though it was still a bit bloodshot and she was flushed, and she was happy to go by herself. I wrote a note describing her symptoms for her GP because there was no physical evidence any more, and mentioned that I thought it could potentially be a cluster headache (many GPs at the time didn't know they were a separate form of headache).

Rachel came back in to see me a couple of days later. She seemed much brighter, if a bit tired. Her doctor had seen her immediately and checked for other nefarious causes, such as stroke, and he had also arranged for her to have an MRI to rule out severe neck damage or an aneurysm (*see* p. 6).

How cluster headaches are treated

Treatment of cluster headaches since their acceptance as a headache distinct from migraine has been haphazard, and mainly applied through the myopia of which aspect of the body's physiology was thought to cause it. For example, Horton (of Horton's Histamine Headache fame) thought that if the histamine response, whatever the trigger, was excessive, he should be able to desensitise the patient through discrete exposure to histamine and that this would have clinical benefits. We see this as a treatment for people with allergies today in which small amounts of the trigger are given to the patient over time to retrain the immune response to something more proportional. However, Horton's trials of desensitising patients to histamine proved ineffective on the whole. He also tried ergotamine, a substance extracted from fungi that has vasoconstrictor effects, but was faced with the issue that it also results in some side effects, including muscle weakness or vision problems. Marcello Fanciullacci had some success with a hospitalised patient who in addition to histamine was administered a cocktail of antihistamines (which seems counterintuitive) and ergotamine to prevent the vasodilatory response of the histamine. Marcello tacitly admits that his desensitisation methodology 'effected by a physician in whom [the patient] had complete confidence and reassurance ... may have had the same effect in alleviating his headache for some time.' Sounds like a placebo effect to me, and indeed did not stand up to later controlled trials involving multiple patients. Antihistamine drugs also proved ineffective as a treatment over a number of controlled trials. So, it is fair to say that mitigating the effects of cluster headache through histamine alone doesn't work.

When Rachel visited the GP surgery on the afternoon she had the headache, the practice nurse administered oxygen as she was by this point feeling the pain come on again. Oxygen has long been used as a treatment for cluster headache; it was first reported in scientific journals in 1981 by Californian Lee Kudrow, father of actress Lisa Kudrow[8] (who played Phoebe in *Friends*), both of whom are sufferers of cluster headache. A further study in support of the use of oxygen was reported by polymath Lance Fogan in 1985, also working out of California.[9] Nowadays, the accepted treatment is to deliver 12–15 litres (around 3–4 liquid gallons) of pure oxygen gas per minute by mask for 20 minutes. It really wasn't known why this had such a remarkable, restorative and instant effect until 10 years ago, when Simon Ackerman and colleagues from the University of California in San Francisco found that oxygen acts to regulate the parasympathetic facial nerves, which in turn lessens the activation of the trigeminal pathway, calming down the cascade of symptoms out of our control that happen in cluster headache.

Of course, we can't go lugging around oxygen tanks on the off-chance we'll get a headache but thankfully there is a more pharmaceutical approach than was prescribed to Rachel. She was told to take sumatriptan at the first sign of the headache and if it reoccurred within two hours, she was to take it again. This treatment was first developed in the 1990s as a subcutaneous injection but has since been developed into pill form, although this doesn't work for everyone. Steve, the husband of a friend, for example, has experienced three cluster headache episodes in eight years, always in February so far. He always carries a sumatriptan injection with him wherever he goes, except for once on a quick trip to London. As he felt the telltale signs of the headache starting, he realised in horror that he didn't have his injection with him. He could have tried to get an emergency appointment with a doctor or gone to a local hospital emergency room but he knew it would take as much time to do that as it would to get the next train for the two-and-a-half-hour journey home. His instincts screamed at him that this was the thing to do. 'Do not pass Go, do not collect £200,' as he put it, instead heading home to his family and his standby oxygen tank and his injection. But he didn't get there fast enough. Steve's window of opportunity to stop a cluster headache is very small, which is probably why oral tablets don't work for him as even they take too long to break down in his system. On the way home the whole shebang hit him, leaving him for two weeks in a dark room waiting for the storm to pass.

The soothing powers of serotonin

Sumatriptan is a serotonin agonist, which means it acts just like serotonin in the brain. It is vasoactive (affects the diameter of the blood vessels) and works to constrict blood vessels (remember, it is the *dilated* blood vessels that are a major trigger to the trigeminal nerve pain pathways) and decrease the inflammatory response. It works just like ergotamine in this respect but ergotamine is an agonist not just for serotonin but also dopamine and noradrenalin, so its effects are less specific and therefore more prone to causing widespread side effects. Relief can be experienced within 10 minutes of ingesting sumatriptan, and is often accompanied by a sensory wave of well-being, thanks to the activation of the happy hormone network. The use of sumatriptan is therefore tightly controlled to ward off addiction and although it is available over the counter, it is only sold in small quantities.

We know that serotonin and melatonin work in balance with each other: as we get sleepy, serotonin is converted into melatonin by the pineal gland. Melatonin production is decreased in cluster headache sufferers both during active cluster periods and in remission, but this is particularly marked during a cluster bout. It may be that there is a problem converting serotonin into melatonin, but it is more likely, given the rhythmicity of the onset of the headache, that the fault lies with serotonin. If there is not enough serotonin, it will have a negative knock-on effect on concentrations of melatonin. There is simply not enough serotonin to convert to change the melatonin concentration. However, using sumatriptan as a pre-emptive strike does not seem to affect the number of headaches people experience. As the drug only acts on one serotonin receptor (there are many) it may be that its effects are too narrow to engender systemic change.

How can we increase the serotonin in our systems?

- Happiness is the key for long-term regulation of serotonin. Without serotonin, we are not happy, and a lack of it is the biggest indicator of depression. The more joyful and happy experiences we have in our lives, the greater the amount of serotonin we produce. Unless we are very depleted, serotonin is quite regulated by our behaviour.
- Light therapy may also be used to increase serotonin levels in the long term (although that would be quite uncomfortable *during* a headache).

The option to medicate

Taking lithium has widespread effects in the brain, but it has also been proven to be effective in the treatment of cluster headache. In experiments conducted by Lee Kudrow, lithium showed dramatic effects in the recurrence of cluster headaches in 27 of 28 patients, meaning it could be used as a preventative measure. We could link this to the now known effects of lithium on the hypothalamus, particularly in the sleep–wake centre, on boosting serotonin concentrations and indeed its action in the preoptic nucleus (*see* p. 100) for sex hormone release. The problem with lithium, however, is that patients often adapt to their doses and require increased amounts to prevent headache episodes, thus leading to undesirable side effects ranging from blurred vision, through balance problems, to full-on convulsions.

Another possible treatment comes from using a cardiac drug called Verapamil, which acts by reducing vasodilation in blood vessels but also affects the hypothalamus itself. Although there are side effects, including constipation and dizziness, Verapamil is better tolerated than lithium and has been shown to be effective in clinical trials for cluster headache. However, careful attention must be paid to patients prescribed this drug due to its effects on the heart. Such monitoring should never end; our life circumstances never stop changing and our physiology is bound up in that so why would we expect the action of drugs we are taking to be constant? Effective treatment of the acute phase of the cluster headache is therefore preferable in most cases.

Chocolate, sex and coffee

For swift serotonin shots, chocolate, which is full of tryptophan, which is then broken down into serotonin, is a good treatment. Sex also results in an injection of serotonin. The case of two male episodic cluster headache sufferers, one of whom was 61 and the other of whom was 47, was reported by Marc Gotkine and colleagues in Israel in 2006. At the point of orgasm with their respective partners, the men reported that their headaches suddenly disappeared. This is somewhat at odds with an earlier report in 1989 by Michael Maliszewski, from Diamond Headache Clinic in Chicago, USA, that sex can *bring on* a cluster headache. However, it should be noted that numbers in this study were very small. Sex headaches in general happen in 1 per cent of people and in more men than women. They occur mainly due to spikes in blood pressure and vasodilation in the head and neck.

Sex is a huge neuroendocrine undertaking. A lot happens – and it is all controlled ultimately by the hypothalamus. So, rebalancing hormonal concentrations through our behaviours can help with the function of these crucial yet unsung regions, and can certainly induce restorative vasoconstriction when in the midst of a headache.

Caffeine is also a vasoconstrictor, which, as we've already learned, is why it is packaged in the same pill as paracetamol, for example. All of this leads us to the conclusion that when in the throes of a cluster headache, the simplest approach to self-medication would be sex with a post-coital snack of coffee and chocolate. Maybe tonight then, dear … but only if there is testosterone to spare.

6

What's a Migraine?

NOT EVERY REALLY PAINFUL headache is a migraine, in much the same way that a really bad cold is not the 'flu. Unless you're a man of course (*see* p. 100 – the theoretical implication of your bigger preoptic nucleus aside, gentlemen). Influenza is an entirely different animal, as those of you who have actually experienced it will know. Migraine, too, has a specific symptom set that means it is recognised now as something totally separate from other classes of headache. Over the next two chapters, we will investigate these symptoms to understand what is going on to create them and how our body reacts to them.

Migraine falls into two-and-a-half categories. You can have 'migraine with aura', which is called 'classic migraine', or 'migraine without aura', which is 'common migraine'. I have experienced both on occasion myself. You can also have 'ocular migraine', which is the aura bit without the pain part – you might just jump straight to feeling groggy, which is why I call it half a category. However, as we shall see, the four component stages that make up a migraine are somewhat shared across these types.

The most interesting aspect of migraine is that it is *an experience that goes beyond the headache component*. It is not just a headache, it is a phenomenological event that comprises four distinct phases:

1 The prodrome phase
2 The aura
3 The pain phase
4 The postdrome phase.

It is important to understand each because this tells us something new about what's going on in our brain to cause them, and also opens windows on how we might be able to solve them.

Something wicked this way comes – the prodrome phase

I have spoken to many migraine sufferers in my time and have learned a lot. However, the most fundamental thing I have discovered is that migraineurs (as we refer to migraine sufferers in the biz) are quite bad at spotting the first stage of migraine: the 'prodrome' phase. As a case in point, I met a 25-year-old man called David and his mum at a headache event once and witnessed a rather heated exchange about this very thing. David's mum swore that she could spot his migraine before he could. 'With every respect, Mum,' and you just *know* the tone of what's coming next is going to be laced with disrespect, 'I think *I*, of *all* people, would know when I am getting a headache, after all.' I interjected (unhelpfully for David) that the last person to know is often the migraineur themselves. Indeed, there is hard, albeit recent, evidence to support this. Ana Gago-Veiga from the Headache Unit in Sanitaria Hospital, Madrid, Spain, worked out that only around a third of patients she surveyed could be classified as good predictors – in that they could spot an impending migraine more than 50 per cent of the time. Even then, it was only because their prodrome symptoms were quite obvious, including pronounced yawning, drowsiness, food craving, adversity to light, increased thirst or blurred vision. Having explained all of this to David, and his rather rapt mum, he sheepishly reported that he had never put these symptoms together with his migraine before. 'I had,' his mum announced, rather too triumphantly, I thought. But it just goes to show: mums really are always right.

As we now know, it takes a certain amount of self-awareness to spot the first stage, the prodrome phase. In this premonitory (something that predicts something bad is about to happen) phase you may be displaying a bunch of behaviours related to the changes that are happening in your brain, and these can occur a couple of days or hours before the migraine starts properly. You might yawn more than usual, be less alert – or even drowsy – have cravings or be hungrier than usual. Walking into shops with really bright mirrored lighting might unsettle you to the point of distraction. These symptoms should not be underestimated.

For the past 10 years, Peter Goadsby from King's College London and some others have been talking about the value of tracking these symptoms to their underlying biology. It's the changes that happen in your brain that sometimes causes the behaviour that we think of as being 'triggers' for migraine. We have to unpack this; ultimately, I am interested in why we have these symptoms. Are these behaviours in some way generated to redress some neurochemical balance that is out of kilter in our brain?

How can we manage this to stop the migraine from going any further? Here's what we know so far.

Yawning chasm

Let's start with yawning. Yawning is an interesting behaviour as it is both physiological and psychosocial. It's very easy to 'catch' a yawn – there have even been studies that have linked exactly how easy you find this to how empathic you are. Well, I am yawning my head off writing this so take from that what you will, and if you feel the urge to yawn right now, go ahead, I won't judge. The reason why we yawn together is because it engenders group alertness; yawning introduces a big dose of oxygen to the body, a fair amount of which reaches your brain, helping you feel more refreshed (which is why we also yawn when we are tired). Evolutionarily, this may have been important when the group was off hunting a woolly mammoth or something; nowadays, military parachutists often report having a jolly good group yawn before they jump out of the plane. (Although between you and me I think yawning might be further down the list of the many functions my body would perform all by itself in this instance.)

It isn't all about the shot of oxygen, though. In 2007, father-and-son duo Andrew and Gordon Gallup from New York State University put cool packs on people's foreheads as they watched videos of people yawning. They discovered that people yawned much less frequently when the cool packs were there, so this indicates that yawning helps cool our brains too; if our head is already cool, we don't catch a yawn as easily. This cooling may help us feel more alert, independent of the extra oxygen. And perhaps the cooling is interacting with a neural pathway that is active in yawning, stifling it for us.

Yawning is an unconscious or automatic behaviour that originates in the brainstem, where lots of species-specific behaviours, such as grooming, originate. So, yawning may be triggered as a thermoregulatory response (we're too hot) or to introduce more oxygen into the brain, which might lead us to think that in the pre-migraine state, the brain is inflamed in some way that increased its local temperature and/or that it is somewhat oxygen depleted. Yawning is our way of self-medicating to reduce that inflammation and increase the oxygen levels.

This relates to neurochemistry in a very specific way through the action of dopamine. Dopamine is one of the main excitatory neurotransmitters in the brain, important in alertness but also movement and how rewarded we feel having behaved in ways that keep us alive (like eating and drinking, and sex, although that is not classed as a behaviour that keeps us alive). Dopamine neurons trigger the act of yawning by causing the hypothalamus to act on the brainstem to carry out the act of yawning itself. In this way, dopamine induces a behaviour to improve our alertness. We know that chemicals that act like dopamine in the brain can cause yawning, and that people with dopamine deficiencies, such as Parkinson's disease patients, yawn less. Because of this, the prevailing wisdom is that higher levels of dopamine cause the symptoms seen in migraine. But the story is more nuanced than that, with the migraineur's *sensitivity to dopamine* being the key issue; migraineurs seem to be particularly sensitive to dopamine concentrations.

There is another view, however. Building on the knowledge that people prone to migraine are hypersensitive to dopamine, Piero Barbanti, the head of the Italian Headache Society, and his colleagues from San Raffaele

Hospital in Rome, Italy, have developed another somewhat complementary idea. Piero has a theory that lower amounts of dopamine, not more, kick off the prodrome symptoms of migraine. I can buy this theory because lower dopamine would have a depressive effect on the brain and so yawning could be instigated to wake the brain up. What happens next, Piero explains, is that the dopamine levels are regulated by the hypothalamus, which takes emergency steps to keep all levels of hormones and neurotransmitters within strict confines. The quick boost of dopamine it administers into the system causes the nausea that is then seen in the next stage of migraine. In experiments where subjects are given a dopamine agonist (that acts just like dopamine in the body) a very small amount induces yawning in migraineurs, whereas those who *don't* get migraine have to take a lot more to have that happen. With increasing dosage, a control person is merely yawning, whereas people who get migraines are by now throwing up all over the place because they are so much more sensitive to it.

How do we reconcile these two theories? The common point here is the migraineurs' sensitivity to dopamine, whether the concentration of dopamine needed to cause the symptoms of the prodrome phase is low or high. You might ask why we care about what causes the migraine symptoms at a neurobiological level, but understanding this might be a way of stopping migraines from happening in the first place. For instance, we can link dopamine to how we feel and we can manipulate it through our behaviours. It makes you think of all the times when you might have unwittingly done something to head off a migraine by boosting your dopamine levels, by giving yourself a rewarding experience like eating something you fancy or having an orgasm. Unfortunately, we'll never know what these behaviours were. This is one of the things we know we don't know – it's fairly impossible to get evidence for what we did in order *not* to experience an event.

It is a bit of a conundrum though, because dopamine is a good mediator of pain, blocking the signal from the trigeminal pain pathway to the brain. But of course the problem is not caused by dopamine alone; dopamine works hand in hand with serotonin – serotonin improves the action of dopamine – with receptors for both often located together. So another argument is that dopamine may not be doing its job properly because serotonin is low, and any regulatory boost the hypothalamus tries to implement is just too late to stop the pain cascade.

Craving a cure?

It is not just yawning that is a striking symptom in the prodrome phase. Changes in appetite are, too. Some people experience a loss of appetite before a headache hits, whereas others crave certain foods, generally of the sweet variety. As we know, appetite is also controlled by the hypothalamus, and a strong hormonal suspect in the latest migraine research is neuropeptide Y, which is a kind of neurotransmitter just like dopamine is. It turns out that orexin (a hormone we met in Chapter 5) also directly interacts with neuropeptide Y (NPY) and so it is implicated as well. Orexin makes us crave specific foods, and when we put this together with our knowledge of prodrome migraine behaviour, it explains why people turn to cheese or chocolate or sometimes high-carbohydrate meals in this phase. That doesn't mean the chocolate is a *trigger* of your headache though; the changes in your brain chemistry are the trigger. We have to be really careful about this: laying off chocolate will not prevent headaches. The changes of activity in your hypothalamus that precede the headache are directly influencing your dietary choices.

Can these cravings tell us anything about what our bodies are lacking? Is our brain pulling our strings to self-medicate us? Migraineurs are generally attracted to sweet foods that will quickly break down into sugar in the body. This might mean that a period of poor diet or irregular eating patterns has led to a hormone imbalance in the hypothalamus, which it is now encouraging you to replenish. It could also be a way to take in energy to help you cope with what is to come (the migraine). Either way, our hypothalamus keeps us in such tight homeostatic control that it is hard to believe that the specific craving that we have has no correlation with what is wrong, and what is causing the headache.

Perhaps understanding what is happening with our hormone levels will help us? Our normal appetite control is a complicated dance between the action of orexin on NPY neurons and vice versa, in addition to the circulating levels of the hormone leptin that is released from fat cells to inhibit hunger. If the level of one of these hormone levels falls, then that affects the action of the others. For example, high leptin leads to a decrease in NPY through the action of orexin, thus discouraging further feeding, and low leptin does the opposite. But the orexin–NPY axis can work outside of the influence of leptin (remember how easy it is to override how full you feel when you absolutely *have* to have dessert?).

Alas, the link between levels of these hormones and the incidence of migraine is befuddled across the scientific literature. Migraine incidence has been linked to low levels of NPY at least in younger patients during the prodrome phase. Levels jumped as the pain phase took over. Orexin levels seem to be low in people who experience episodic migraines (which would theoretically lead to a loss of appetite) and high in those who have a chronic variety (those who get cravings).

More evidence about the role of orexin comes from those who experience the sleep disturbance narcolepsy, or uncontrolled falling asleep. This is caused by a loss of orexin neurons in the hypothalamus and such patients report at least a doubling of migraine prevalence in comparison with non-narcoleptics, boosting the evidence that low orexin is a driving factor in migraine. But as with cluster headache, the critical factor may not be the actual concentrations of orexin but rather *our sensitivity to it.*

How this might manifest itself in real life can explain the cravings. We know that orexin itself can cause specific cravings, but if NPY isn't there to control the appetite, then the craving will be unleashed. As the pain phase of the headache takes hold, the levels of NPY increase because just like dopamine, it is a powerful painkiller in the trigeminal pathway and also causes constriction in the vasculature of the head. And just like dopamine, this higher concentration boost happens *too late* to stop the pain from starting.

The clearest things we can say are that these hormones are implicated somehow in the disordered physiology, or pathophysiology, of the migraine and have the power to manipulate our behaviour. Directly affecting the action of these chemicals medically is a possible pathway to intervention.

A chemical conundrum

So we now know that dopamine, serotonin and neuropeptide Y all lead to that feeling that something is not quite right through their actions, and can make us agitated and cranky. This discomfort or dissonance with what is going on around you is no doubt linked to dips in serotonin levels as well as oxytocin. Even outside of headache, our levels of these hormones peak and trough throughout our lives and are quite dependant on what life has bestowed upon us, or indeed hit us with. Serotonin in our story is consistent with chocolate craving; packed with tryptophan, which is converted into serotonin in our bodies, chocolatey goodness is bound to prop up our concentrations.

Oxytocin, meanwhile, is the bonding hormone, released in large amounts in females after giving birth – and postnatal women report a much lower incidence of migraine. Individuals of both sexes experience a boost in oxytocin in the early days of a love affair, too. It helps people become somewhat addicted to each other, making them feel uncomfortable when they are apart from their amour. This explains why new affairs eschew the involvement of others that might compete with the attentions of the lovers, hence all previous friends are dropped like hot potatoes. It doesn't last though; levels normalise, there is time once again for friends, and being with your partner is not as big a deal. Sorry for reducing such a wonderful human experience to the specific action of a hormone – of course it is just a little more complicated, but here is my point: if your oxytocin dips, how does that make you feel?

Migraine sufferers in the prodrome phase feel disconnected; I have heard many use the phrase 'I just feel needy'. This feeling should never be ignored as it is *entirely* related to low oxytocin. Hugs to the rescue! Even having some time alone with a loved one's undivided attention or telling a loved one how you feel about them, and why, helps to boost their oxytocin levels (e.g. you clean the bathroom, you make nice risotto, your smile fills me up ... feel free to improvise) and yours will get a nice bump too. Sex helps, but only with partners with whom there is an emotional connection (although serotonin and dopamine don't mind so much about that). This all matters because there are loads of oxytocin receptors on the trigeminal pathway neurons and if oxytocin binds with them, the trigeminal neuron can't pass on its signal. In other words, if the oxytocin receptors are not fed, then the pain signals pass at full power to the brain. Low oxytocin is therefore a big problem for the migraineur. Choose a hugger as your partner; they don't call it [neuro]chemistry for nuthin'!

Do you see what I see? The aura

After the prodrome phase we have a bit of a divergence. Some people go straight to the pain phase and this is called 'common migraine', but some have another step: the migraine aura, turning their experience into what we refer to as 'classic migraine'. I have spoken to many people about their experience of the migraine aura, but actually, of the migraine population, only 20 per cent have experienced an aura. They may have experienced one or two in their lifetime or they may experience them every time they have an episode of migraine. And then there are those who experience this stage without going on to the pain phase of migraine – theirs is called 'ocular migraine'. This name flags up the most common form of aura, which is a visual disturbance.

Ben was a 22-year-old PhD student when he experienced his first aura. It was a Sunday morning, and he had to go into the university to do some writing for his thesis. He didn't really want to because he had felt 'fuggy' for the previous couple of days, but he hadn't got as much done as he had wanted to that week so he was giving it another push to reach his target. It was a sunny, fresh spring day, the best time for clearing his head. Ben remembers smiling to himself as he put the key in his office door; he was thinking this might be the first beer garden afternoon of the year if he could get finished up by three. And then the door disappeared.

I asked him if this came as a shock. He looked at me as if I had 16 heads. 'Well, of course; that didn't usually happen.' After a couple of moments just staring at where the door should be, Ben realised the whole door hadn't disappeared, just the part with the door handle and the key, and that this was in his peripheral vision as he was looking straight ahead at the name plate mounted on the door. He cautiously moved his eyes around and realised that the 'hole', which scientists and clinicians call a 'scotoma', was in the same place in his peripheral vision no matter where his eyes were pointed, and he couldn't see whatever fell into the hole.

What's interesting about Ben's report is the sudden onset, and it went away just as quickly – by the time he had managed to sit down at his desk to gather his thoughts, it was gone. He experienced it for five minutes, tops. Most people who report aura can detect the onset as a gradual change in their perceptions. It usually lasts between 5 and 20 minutes and is undetectable after an hour. Just like Ben, most people are completely freaked out by their first experience and whether or not it is followed up by a headache, it is well worth talking to a clinician about it, and certainly if the aura lasts for more than an hour.

If we put all of the ways people experience aura together, a pattern soon emerges. In their simplest forms, visual auras are composed of phosphenes – our perception of spots of light that aren't really there. You can induce your own phosphenes easily by pushing on your eyeball gently, close your eyes first! That spot of light is caused because you have activated the retina mechanically through the pressure you've put on the eye. Because the retina has been activated, the brain 'perceives' light, even though it is illusory. You can induce phosphenes by activating the part of the brain that decodes the electrical signals coming from the retina, too. In the 1930s, Wilder Penfield from McGill University would send electrical currents into the open brains of conscious patients he was operating on in order to see what different parts did. If the bit he stimulated was important in arm movements, the patient's arm would move. If it detected light in a specific part of the visual field, the patient would see a phosphene there. Wilder managed to make many amazingly useful maps of the function of different parts of the brain in this way. You might think this sounds barbaric, but even in the 1930s it was possible to operate on conscious patients under just local anaesthetic. Indeed, it was preferable, as it guided neurosurgeons to areas of vital importance for life, such as speech areas, or movement regions, so that they could be spared if possible. It is a practice still continued today, although scientific investigation is less invasive now. By sending magnetic pulses into your brain, I can activate the neurons that make your body move, or that make you see a phosphene. Called transcranial magnetic stimulation, it is a great tool to gently and reversibly switch on bits of your brain so that we can know exactly what it is doing, and when.

Scientifically induced phosphenes can be obvious. They are like flashes of light against a black background, or more subtle changes in quality of the resolution of your vision in an area of your visual field. In a migraine aura, there is more structure. When you are perceiving a phosphene, it obscures what you should really be seeing at that point in your visual field and so you are essentially blind in that area. American psychologist Karl Lashley experienced aura himself, and was interested in what was happening in his brain to cause these perceptions.

What Karl realised in 1941 was that while your earliest perception may be a small spot (easily overlooked by the visual system) it seems to expand, and the shape of the scotoma never changes, it just gets bigger. He linked this to how electrical activity might be spreading over the area of the visual system in the brain; the earliest area (V1, also known as primary visual cortex and also striate cortex because of how it looks under a microscope) is important in perceiving lines, hence the perception of zigzags made of straight lines. More advanced areas in the visual system catch light from much bigger areas in the visual field and so stimulation there will cause a much bigger scotoma. If the electricity is passed in a non-random way, the scotoma will hold its shape and merely appear to be expanding. The edges of the scotoma, or the 'fortifications' as they are called, do not expand, but are duplicated to fit the bigger shape and there seems to be a scintillation across the levels of boundaries, 'like the illusion of movement of a revolving screw'. When he compared notes this seemed to be common for all observers. Karl was onto something. By plotting the rate of enlargement of his scotoma, the rate of the scintillation (about 10 waves per second) and putting that together with what he knew about how the visual cortex propagates the electrical signal, he concluded that the two were related, and at least in his case, this wave of excitation in his brain must be travelling at a rate of 3mm (0.12in) per minute.

These 'ripple-waves in the cerebral pond' had already been suggested in 1904 by a British neurologist Sir William Gowers, but without precise neurological insight at the time, he proposed them more as a metaphor to understand the phenomenon. Now, Karl had added some observational heft to the story. But at the time, the neurological community was consumed by the idea that each bit of the brain did one thing, or 'functional localisation' as we still call it, and wasn't interested in hearing how waves of activity could pass between one area and another resulting in complex perceptions and behavioural effects. It took until 1990 and Gregory Barkley's team in Wayne State University, Detroit, Michigan, to definitively visualise these waves in the brain of patients experiencing migraine aura using a technique called magnetoencephalography (MEG) (*see* p. 201), which detects the magnetic fields emanating from your head, an indicator of the electrical activity that is going on inside your skull.

Other types of aura

Yet aura is not just a visual issue. The next most common type is sensory aura, which takes the form of a creeping tingling in your skin, sometimes over the head and sometimes in the limbs. It can make your skin hypersensitive and even present as a dull response in your limbs to movement, or paralysis. As with visual disturbance, it's always important to go to a medical professional the first time you experience this to rule out other causes such as stroke. Somatosensory tingling during aura is not to be mixed up with Autonomous Sensory Meridian Response (ASMR), which is also described as a tingling over the head and neck after triggers such as repetitive movements or whispering.

Although it is relatively new to scientific enquiry, there is already a multimillion-pound YouTube cottage industry trying to induce that pleasurable feeling some people describe as a brain orgasm. Because of this, there has been much interest in trying to induce it as a happiness boost in depression and other affective disorders. Most research to date focuses on pleasant inducement of the ASMR effect, although there have been some reports of ASMR occurring when people view particularly violent scenes. It certainly needs more investigation, if not just to understand any commonalities that may exist between ASMR and somatosensory aura in migraine. For instance, Nick Davis from Manchester Metropolitan University and his team have shown that background music stops ASMR from happening, so that distraction from another modality (in this case hearing) stops a somatosensory effect. Can we mine this knowledge to minimise the effect of migraine aura?

It is even possible to have other sensory auras including olfactory (smelling something that isn't there or extra sensitivity to smell), auditory (hearing dripping taps, loss of hearing, tinnitus or extra sensitivity to sound) and taste (particularly manifesting as a metallic taste in your mouth). Interestingly, these are also symptoms often reported in geriatric patients suffering from urinary tract (and particularly kidney) infections that have caused severe dehydration.

Aura can therefore manifest itself in any of our sensory systems but we have left one out. Everybody thinks about the five senses: seeing, hearing, taste, smell, touch. But touch is a very specific term; it would be better to use a more umbrella term such as somatosensation, which encompasses both touch and also our *awareness of where our body is in space*. It is this 'proprioception' that can also be disturbed by aura, leading to a certain clumsiness. Some of us just have this all the time unfortunately, and have the broken nose to prove it.

We now know that there is a clearly defined pattern of activity in the brain that occurs during the aura that causes these sensory effects, independent of outside stimuli. Work to define the migraine aura intensified in the 1990s after Sir William Gower and Karl Lashley's suggested 'ripple-waves' were seen using MEG.

It turns out that what you are observing during aura is a wave of excitation across your cortex. In this wave, many neurons become active in a coordinated way and this electrical activity travels as a surge. This is what causes the sensory disturbance, as brain cells are active and usually their activation is because you are sensing something; so you see things that aren't really there, feel touch when you are not being touched, etc. However, crucially, this wave of excitation is followed by a wave of depression called 'cortical spreading depression', where your neurons go completely asleep or more properly, become inactive. This is the big picture of how the abnormal pattern of electrical activity affects your behaviour in migraine and kicks off the pain. But what is happening to create this activity?

This is important, because some of the causes of migraine interact directly with a particular phenomenon at the level of the cell that is happening in all of us, all of the time! I'm referring to what makes you tick – quite literally, because that's how this phenomenon sounds to our ears when amplified in the lab! If you listen to the electrical activity in a single neuron it sounds like static noise over a radio. Slow it right down and you can hear every crackle, every tick. Each one of those ticks is called an *action potential*, a little pulse of electricity passing down that neuron, a signal, a *nerve impulse*, each one lasting about a millisecond. It is well named because it truly represents your potential for action. For you to be able to think, walk, watch television, read

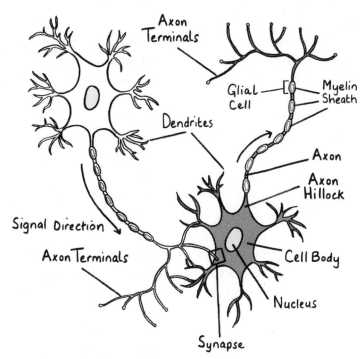

FIGURE 3 Two Neurons 'Talking'

this book or do anything at all, you need millions of these ticks in just the right places in your brain at just the right times. And it's all going on without you even knowing it's there.

It's really worth looking at how action potentials are made so that we can find out how these waves of excitation kick off the pain we experience in migraine.

How do you tick?

You might remember from school that electricity is all about the movement of charged particles. In the body, these are ions like sodium (with its chemical name Na^+) and potassium (K^+). When the neuron is not doing anything and resting, there are many more negative particles on the inside of the neuron than the outside. These nerve cells are really particular about what comes in and goes out and have little doors made out of protein in their membrane that only open for a particular thing, like a gate that only lets sodium in and out, for example. Whether these gates (called ion channels) are open or closed depends on how negative the inside of the cell is. If there is a little spark of electricity, that might have come from another neuron (we'll talk about this soon), or a feather brushing your arm or some other sensory stimulus, these gates open and ions like sodium move in. Sodium is a positive ion and it wants to rush into the neuron because there isn't much there already. Also, the inside of the neuron is very negative, so because opposites attract the positive sodium ions are drawn there. So, very rapidly the inside of the cell gets even more positive than the outside was, and this flip in polarity is the first part of the action potential and is called depolarisation. For the sparkier among you, it is about a 110mv difference (from -70mv to +40mv).

Now we have to get the neuron back to normal resting state again because until it is back to resting state, it can't generate another signal. Because the inside is more positive at this point, the gates for sodium shut. It's trapped! But when the inside is this positive, the gates for potassium open. Potassium is also a positive ion and is usually much more concentrated inside the cell than outside the cell. It leaves the neuron, fast, because the outside is more negative now and opposites attract, and there is not much potassium out there so it wants to populate it. In a fraction of a blink, the upswing of the pulse has been turned back down again. The action potential is done and this part of the cell is repolarised, back to having the inside more negative again. It even has an extra dip in negativity to finish with a flourish before it gets to the normal resting state. The neuron sets about kicking all that sodium out again by a kind of ion prisoner exchange, using a protein in the membrane that pumps out three sodium ions for every two potassium ions it lets in.

Anything that blocks the way ions move into or out of the cell through the ion channels, or plays with the concentration of ions, will mess with this entire process, and *there will be consequences*. For example, the wave of excitation in migraine will cause potassium to get trapped on the outside of the cell, and this activates pain receptors in the blood vessels – not good for us migraine sufferers. More on this later too.

The role of axons

The action potential is kicked off in the cell body of a neuron, in an area called the axon hillock just at the start of the axon (or in less technical terms, 'the stringy bit') that carries the signal to the next neuron. If we think about one neuron in particular, there will be many neurons connecting to it trying to pass on their signals. It is the axon hillock's job to decide if it has had enough excitatory input to pass on the signal. If it has, then it generates an action potential. If it hasn't then it just keeps quiet.

Some other things are worth saying that are important for our cortical spreading depression story. Action potentials are all-or-nothing events. They all look exactly the same. You can't add them together. So how do you know if there is a particularly forceful stimulus for example, or a really bright light as opposed to a dim one? Well, magnitude is transmitted by frequency. A little touch will elicit a few action potentials per unit time, but a proper punch will cause loads of action potentials. You also can't have two action potentials in the same patch of neurons at the same time because the ions are in the wrong place to generate one. And action potentials travel in one direction only, away from the cell body. The extra dip in negativity of the inside of the cell when potassium has flooded out takes care of that detail.

The action potential travels down the axon by regenerating itself at every point down the neuron. Support cells called glial cells wrap themselves around most neurons, forming a myelin sheath that acts like the insulation we see on electrical cable. The action potential can then jump between gaps between the glial cells and only has to regenerate itself every now and again. This makes nerve conduction faster and more efficient. We can track rates of myelination (the creation of the myelin sheath) in different parts of the brain to the acquisition of new skills in babies and young people.[1]

The case of Golgi vs Cajal

Because we are living human beings and don't catch excitability from some neuroscientist in a lab coat with an electrode stuck into the Petri dish in which we are living (although there is a movie in that), we have to think about how it happens in real life, where neurons don't live in isolation. Let's think about two neurons. How does activity in the first get passed on to the second? This fundamental question caused one of the biggest and certainly most infamous tiffs in scientific history. It started when the Italian Camillo Golgi developed a way to see the structure of a neuron and what was in it under the rudimentary microscopes that were around in the mid- to late-1800s. He would slice up brain tissue as thinly as he could, shine light through the material and magnify the image through a number of convex lenses. However, brain tissue is translucent, and so he had to develop a silver substance to wash the brain tissue in. The silver particles would stain the individual neurons black and show very fine details of what they looked like and where they went, which led Golgi to describe them as an interconnected series of 'tubes'.

Soon after, the Spanish neuroanatomist Santiago Ramón Y Cajal refined Golgi's technique and discovered that neurons are discrete entities in and of themselves. He also linked age to what the neurons he could see looked like, with their form becoming much more complex with maturity.

Golgi was furious, and diametrically opposed to Cajal's views; Golgi believed that the nerve cells he could see acted much like the blood vessels in the body, whereas Cajal correctly identified that they were separate, with gaps in between them that had their own functions, not just acting like transit stations in a network. In recognition of their work, both Cajal and Golgi won the Nobel Prize in Physiology or Medicine in 1906. Awkward.

The drama didn't end there. Both anatomists used their acceptance speeches in Sweden to attack the other's view, leading to quite fractious scenes and a definite sense of unease in the auditorium. Probably just as well they hadn't won the Nobel Peace Prize, although there was no way that was in either of their futures. Of the two, Cajal was the more magnanimous, acknowledging that if it hadn't been for Golgi, he could not have made his own discovery. Golgi was bound by his education and the prevailing views at the time, whereas he, Cajal, had the kind of mind that could look beyond current wisdom to interpret what they could both see in a different, and ultimately more prescient, way.

Bridging the gap

The gap between nerve cells is called the synapse and provides a bit of a problem for our conduction of our action potential; the electrical signal can't jump this kind of fissure. What seems like a complicated system, however, allows for a really discrete way to control excitability in the brain. Instead of nerve conduction being entirely electrical, the synapse introduces a chemical component. The arrival of the action potential at the end of the neuron, called the terminal bouton, opens up calcium ion channels in the terminal or presynaptic (before the synapse) membrane. Calcium comes into the neuron and binds with little pouches or vesicles full of neurotransmitters such as glutamate or the dopamine and serotonin that we have already met. The vesicles bind with the presynaptic membrane and the contents are dumped out into the synapse. It is the neurotransmitters that lock onto specific receptors in the membrane of the next neuron (postsynaptic membrane) to open ion channels specific for either excitatory (positive ions such as sodium) or inhibitory (negative ions such as chloride) inputs. The axon hillock then decides whether or not there is enough net excitation to start off an action potential in the second (or postsynaptic) neuron. If there isn't enough, then an action potential simply isn't generated.

Wave action

In the traditionally called 'cortical spreading depression', the first step is a wave of excitation, so it has now been renamed 'cortical spreading depolarisation'. This is a huge and co-ordinated excitation that radiates from a point in the cortex, most regularly being in the visual cortex (this is situated at the very back of your brain and is the first place the electrical signal that is made in your eyes in response to light goes). Literally every cell is depolarised and active at the same time, it's a brainstorm. It is also very like the brain activity seen in epilepsy.

The link between epilepsy and migraines

Epilepsy, from the Greek *epi-* or 'upon' and *-lepis'* meaning 'taking hold of' or 'grasping', is diagnosed after two such seizures. The abnormal brain activity in epilepsy usually begins in a small area of cortex that is damaged or malfunctioning in some way. Very often, it begins in the temporal lobe, the area of the brain that processes what objects look like as well as hearing, memory and speech comprehension (in the left hemisphere). This activity in the epileptic brain can cause hallucinations, just as with migraine aura – the experience of seeing something or hearing something that isn't there. The difference between what happens in epilepsy and migraine aura is that in migraine, following the initial activation of neurons, all neural activity stops behind the leading wave; no more action potentials, no more activity at all and so neural activity is completely depressed and, crucially, because of this, there is no epileptic seizure. In epilepsy, the brainstorm continues wave after wave.

Perhaps not surprisingly, there is a genetic link between the two; families with two or more close relatives with epilepsy have been found to also have a prevalence of migraine with aura. The two conditions are genetically similar, but while both are rooted in hyperexcitability, there is a fundamental difference in the receptors that underlie the effect, modulating the behavioural consequences.

The wave of excitability explains the symptoms of the aura, as it slowly passes over the cortex at a rate of around 3mm (0.12in) per minute. It is possible for people to recognise more than one aura; it's not always the case that they only experience a single type, although they do tend to occur sequentially. We can visualise it this way. Let's say that the excitability starts in your occipital cortex at the back of your brain and radiates out from there. Since your occipital cortex is concerned with vision, activity here will cause you to see an aura pattern as described before. When it hits the temporal cortex at the bottom of your brain there may be some auditory or perhaps memory disturbance. The wave will hit the parietal lobe at pretty much the same time, so it is possible to have two symptoms simultaneously, and this is where you might get some tingling, usually on the opposite side to where the wave is passing through your somatosensory cortex.

Wilder Penfield mapped this out using his electro-physiology technique on awake patients who were having brain surgery. He realised that the more sensitive an area of the body, such as the lips or fingertips, the more neurons were devoted to the processing of sensory information from there. Each area of the body has a place in the somatosensory cortex, which lives just before the middle of the brain moving from back to front. If you point to the centre of your head (humans are strangely very accurate when pointing to the centre of their heads!), your somatosensory cortex lies about a finger space behind that and extends down the side of your brain, with sections devoted to all the parts of your body. So as the wave passes by it activates all of these regions.

The wave usually stops at the central 'sulcus' (the big crack that denotes the start of frontal lobe), but if it does pass it immediately encounters the primary motor cortex, which is organised in much the same way as the somatosensory cortex. Again, though, Wilder found that the size of a region devoted to moving part of the body was related to the dexterity we need there, so the area for moving the fingers is much bigger than that for moving the thigh, even though our hands are so much smaller than our thighs. Further forward, our wave finds planning, thinking and emotion centres, which means that as it passes over the frontal cortex, you might feel a bit shaky, clumsy, foggy and generally out of sorts. If the wave gets as far as the very front of your brain your sense of smell and taste will be affected, too. For the wave to traverse the entire brain would take 50 minutes at 3mm (0.12in) per minute for the average 15cm (6in) brain, but up to 30 minutes for the usual half a brain the wave extends to.

However, if the wave doesn't get as far as the frontal cortex then why are these symptoms that come from there so prevalent during the aura? The answer lies in anatomical and functional connectivity between the back of the brain and the front.

I once ran an experiment with a great colleague Alison Lane and a group of other fine people in which we decreased the activity in the back of the brain using electrical stimulation and looked to see what was happening in the whole brain using functional MRI. It turns out that even though we hadn't done anything in the front of the brain, there were a load of regions there where there was less activity than usual. It stands to reason that the wave of excitation and following wave of depression will be having remote effects much further forward than where the wave stops, never mind what is happening under the cortex in the hypothalamus and other areas. But what is driving the complete depression of activity that follows the excitation?

Own goal

It's a little bit like the last minute in a football match when you are 1–0 behind. You only need to draw to win the league but if you lose, you get nothing. Your team throws all of its players forwards, including the goalkeeper. But disaster, your number 11 has a bad touch, loses possession and the other team goes on the break. All of your players are out of position and can't defend against the inevitable goal. If we think of your players as ions, and link this to what happens in the action potential, we've got our explanation.

Our action potentials are fast and furious. Remember that the number of action potentials denote the strength of the response because action potentials are all-or-nothing events. But these continual action potentials put all of the ions that cause the action potential in the wrong place after a while. Sodium rushes in and potassium rushes out, but with continual action potentials the sodium-potassium pump can't redress the balance to a proper resting state where there would be more potassium inside the cell than outside of the cell and more sodium outside than inside. The glial cells can't clear the potassium quickly enough. Since the lowest glial-to-neuron ratio in the brain is found in the visual cortex, this may be why this is the most usual, and first, aura that is experienced. Ultimately, sodium gets trapped on the inside and potassium on the outside, making it impossible to generate an action potential at all! Everything stops.

However, the effects of lots of potassium being in the extracellular space where it doesn't belong are wider than just shutting down the ability to generate action potentials. Potassium acts directly on the tiny branches of the arteries, called arterioles, which then lead to the even tinier capillaries that transfer oxygen and nutrients to the brain tissue as part of the blood–brain barrier. All of the potassium that is floating around the extracellular space acts on the smooth muscle that makes up the wall of the arterioles to constrict the muscle, thereby slowing down the blood flow to that region and reducing the amount of oxygen to the brain tissue, prolonging the depression of neural activity. Because the blood flow is decreased, the high levels of potassium can't be removed efficiently so it hangs around for even longer. As the concentration rises even further, the vasoconstriction gets even more pronounced, perpetuating the cycle that results in the prolonged depression of local activity and 'ischemia' (from the Greek *ishaimos* or 'stopping blood').

This neuronal silence lasts for a few minutes but the recovery to normal activity takes up to 30 minutes. The regional blood flow changes, and the 'hypovolemia' (low blood volume) it causes seems to track the neurological changes seen during cortical spreading depolarisation and the following depression. In 1981 this was named 'spreading oligaemia'[2] by Jes Oleson, a Danish neurologist, one of the first to suggest cortical spreading depression as the mechanism underlying migraine with aura. This was helped in no small part by his decision to set up the Copenhagen Acute Headache Clinic, a place where people in the throes of a headache could come to get some help if they happened to be in Copenhagen, but who also provided valuable data to allow Jes and his colleagues to test their theories. What Jes found was that this hypovolemia spread at the same rate as the neuronal excitability wave, and would continue for 30–60 minutes depending on the patient. Jes observed two other issues:

1 Cortical blood flow continued to be reduced after the aura and during the initial phase of the headache, with patchy increased flow seen up to 2–6 hours later.
2 The side of the headache usually corresponded to the side of the vascular change.

This is excellent evidence to point to potassium as our culprit, because potassium acts directly on the trigeminal pain receptors, or 'noiciceptors', of the arterioles. Therefore, the pain that is generated in the headache phase of the migraine that has been preceded by aura comes from something that happened in the brain and is not purely a vascular issue (as in other headaches). With blood flow reductions of about 20–25 per cent, it's not thought that this is powerful enough to underlie the focal effects of the migraine pain, but it does serve to trap the potassium in situ to do its worst on your noiciceptors and can become critically focused in one place. And what happens when you activate the pain receptors? Your brain thinks you are under threat and arranges a hefty inflammatory response to sort it out, including things we're familiar with by now – prostaglandins, mast cells full of histamine and nitric oxide, all of which will try to induce vasodilation to regulate the blood flow again.

Other changes outside of the cortex are happening, too; the hypothalamus is activated, because it is certainly involved in the autonomic response to threat, and dopamine and neuropeptide Y concentrations increase. The brainstem is cooking because this is where all of the cell bodies of the sensory pain neurons are grouped and activity here is tightly coupled with the hypothalamus through the production of certain proteins that is prompted by the cortical spreading depolarisation and depression. Neuropeptides such as Substance P and nitric oxide as well as calcitonin gene-related peptide (CGRP, more of which on p. 173–5) are released, which perpetuate the inflammatory response in the meninges or the membranes covering the brain and cause vasodilation there. Also, the middle meningeal artery is dilated via the 'trigemino-parasympathetic reflex' – sensory activation of the trigeminal nerve automatically leads to dilation of this blood vessel that feeds much of the back of the brain and brings blood to the frontal regions, too.

This all happens even without the pain signals being perceived by you, in much the same way that if somebody taps just below your kneecap, your leg extends by reflex to protect the tendon there because the tap makes it think it has been stretched.

The aura and what is happening in the brain to underlie these sensory disturbances very clearly explains what then causes the classical migraine pain in a particular place on your head. But hold on, you can have the very same migraine pain without experiencing the aura. Does that mean that common migraine is a purely vascular headache with no underlying brain changes driving the conditions that create the pain (that comes from the blood vessels, as with all other headaches)? Well, Peter Goadsby from King's

College London believes that all migraine headaches start with these activity and chemical changes in the brain. He argues that cortical spreading depolarisation happening is actually happening in the brain of every migraineur, it's just they might not *experience* it as a sensory disturbance. Andrea Harriott from the National Yang-Ming University in Taipei puts it beautifully. It is possible, she says, that some migraine patients without a perceived aura still have the electrical and chemical changes going on in their brains, but that their 'cortical ineloquence stops it from being felt.' It also explains why people like Ben – for whom the door disappeared – has only experienced three auras in his life, although he has had countless migraines in his 44 years on the planet.

What a pain

Migraine pain is particular. True to its original moniker – *hemi* ('half') and *krania* ('skull'), morphing into the word 'migraine' through Late Latin and then French – the pain is felt in one side of the head. It might always be the same side, or even the same spot, but it doesn't have to be. Either way, the pain doesn't usually switch sides, though eventually it may be felt all over the head as the pain phase progresses.

The ubiquitous throbbing pain that migraineurs describe is often centred in the forehead towards the temple but actually can be felt anywhere, but with the very back of the head being the least reported pain zone. (In fact, headaches here perversely often indicate eye strain as this is where most of the early visual processing is done.) The throbbing often appears to follow the heartbeat and indicates the extreme vasodilation that is occurring in the brain.

The demon within

The pain of migraine has been described by cultures for more than 5000 years, going back to the Mesopotamian poems of Sumer and Babylonia, when it was given equal status with the other physiological effects of photophobia (sensitivity to light), nausea, vomiting and a tension in facial features. It's not hard to imagine how this taking over of one's physiological state five millennia ago would have been seen at the time as some form of possession. The finger of blame was pointed at demons, in particular in Mesopotamia and the demon class Asakku,[3] which were held responsible for everything from epilepsy and headache (interesting, now knowing the genetic link they have!) to infectious diseases but that manifested themselves as shivers and chills, jaundice and exhaustion. Migraine was treated with incantations but also trephination, or making a hole in the skull to let the poisoned blood and, of course, the demon out. Archaeology tells us that this was a widespread medical practice from Neolithic times, wherever early humans found themselves, although the justification for it may have changed over time.

Given that migraine has been around for so long, it is rather fascinating that it hasn't been selected out of our genome by evolution if it serves no valuable purpose; there must be some reason why we need it like a hole in our head. We'll come back to this later.

But why do we experience it at least initially in one place? The answer to this lies in our old friend, referred pain. The nerve fibres that carry the pain signals from both the meninges and skin and muscles are all lumped together in one tract, and also can come from a wide area of the brain. It is the same principle whereby pain signals from the heart – perhaps if the heart muscle is not getting enough oxygen – is not perceived by you as a 'pain in your heart' but rather a 'pain in your left arm or jaw'. It's because the sensory nerves from your heart are bound up with the pathway from your arm and jaw, and the brain can't distinguish between them. So in migraine, you feel the pain in one focal place and where that is depends on your anatomy.

The migraine pain signals in the headache phase are created in three ways. The first is the extension of the blood vessel walls themselves, indicating danger. The second thing to think about is that the substances that are causing the inflammation are making the peripheral branches of the trigeminal nerve (and remember, this extends all over the head) much more sensitive to pain than usual. The third problem is that the spinal trigeminal nucleus of the brainstem is in overdrive because those peripheral receptors are going nuts. These activations are passed through connections with the great sorting house of signal known as the thalamus,[4] which sits above the hypothalamus (and is in fact how the *hypo*thalamus gets its name, borrowing from the Greek *hypo* for 'under'), which has anatomical links all over the brain and so explains many of the other symptoms of migraine. Activations from here to the motor cortex make you unable to control your muscles, including, most commonly, those of the face. Attempting to move makes pain even worse because you are trying to make a part of your brain that is already buzzing do something else. You might be clumsy and unable to focus because your parietal cortex is being stimulated (meaning you can't use it for your aims of planning to get from A to B). Somatosensory cortex activation will of course make you feel the pain in your head but it will also make you tingly or numb or even hugely sensitive to touch, to the point where you feel it as pain anywhere in your body. If your temporal cortex goes off then the same will happen with sound. You might have memory loss for a while, too, in addition to being extremely sensitive to odours. The gold standard of course is photophobia, where overactivation of the visual cortex means that any more activation by light sends it into hyperdrive, further perpetuating the pain response. This completes the cacophony of cortical catastrophe (now there's a tongue twister).

The structures that live under the cortex are vulnerable too. For example, the trigeminal nucleus of the brainstem is connected to various areas of the hypothalamus that control the endocrine hormone system as well as the autonomic nervous system of our whole body. So this explains the systemic response of nausea, vomiting and appetite changes. Really interestingly, there is a pathway that extends to the zona incerta, which sits below the thalamus, too. We talked about this region in Chapter 4 because it is an area that we are beginning to understand as being involved in your subjective experience of pain, i.e. it is part of the system that determines your pain threshold. Standing on a Lego brick in your bare feet in the dark is the most unimaginable pain known to humans (OK, we are talking about me here) save for childbirth.

But some people brush it off because they have a high threshold for activation of their zona incerta. Your levels of endogenous opioids, or your body's natural painkillers, are also important in this dance our brain does to decide how bad pain is. But the zona incerta is also involved in chronic pain.

Sameth Eldabe, a world-renowned pain consultant, tells me that people who had spinal surgery in the past because of a trapped nerve, misplaced disk or similar sometimes revisit their clinician years later because their pain symptoms have returned. After tests, the doctor may have to tell them that there is no physical cause for their pain – the spine is fine, nothing is impeded. This is chronic pain. The doctor can only help people cope with the pain. But guess what? Spontaneous activation of the zona incerta is seen at the arrival of the perceived pain. So, we can separate out the sensory component of pain (the somatosensory cortex) and the affective component (the zona incerta). If, as Rodrigo Noseda, a lifetime migraine researcher from Harvard Medical School, says, there is a direct activation of the zona incerta in the migraine, there is an instant mechanism by which any pain will be dialled up in your perception. What a mess! This phase can take from 4 to 72 hours to clear but of course depending on your physiological state before the attack, it could take longer. And it doesn't end there.

It ain't over till it's over – the postdrome phase

Without treatment, this phase of the migraine has to take its course. The brain's natural way of blocking pain – including boosting dopamine, serotonin and natural endorphins (which act like opioid painkillers such as morphine) – will eventually manage to get control and the trigeminal pathways in the brain will calm down, which in turn will stop the nausea through the hypothalamic pathway. And now we enter the postdrome phase. Energy is low, you are mentally foggy. Two plus two might make four but who the heck cares? It is a literal headache hangover, and you had zero fun getting there. Having said that, some people feel euphoric in this phase, which is due to a boost in both the endorphins needed to kill the pain but also the dopamine that has also been released to help block the pain signals.[5]

This 'out-of-whack' or 'zombie-like' feeling is present after the peak pain has passed. Even though the pain is dissipating, the wider hypothalamic functions still need sorting out. Your hormones are all over the place. The length of time your postdrome phase takes is dependent on how disturbed these hormones are and given that it is a very interdependent system and controls most of your bodily functions, it's not hard to see why it has such a widespread effect. Pyari Bose who was doing his PhD with Peter Goadsby at King's College London recently used fMRI (see p. 104) to show that there is a distinct decrease in blood flow around the brain in the postdrome phase, which is hardly surprising in light of the vasoconstrictor brakes the autonomic nervous system had to apply to all those dilated blood vessels! Also, it is unwise to ignore it. Symptoms such as this are trying to tell you something. Mental tiredness means your neurotransmitters need replenishment or rebalancing; rest and sleep help with that. Both mental and physical exhaustion can be helped by introducing a sensible eating pattern with adequate hydration.

Give your body time; it has undergone a pretty spectacular brain event that's affected everything, it has to recover. If you don't, and your hormones and neurotransmitters remain haywire, a migraine will happen again, and sooner than you would wish.

7

What Causes Migraine and What Can We Do About It?

W E SAW IN THE previous chapter that migraine is an all-encompassing brain and body event involving many of the pathways, brain structures, neurotransmitters and hormones that we have seen in other types of headaches. However, migraine is the dark symphony of all of these components working together. With so many factors involved, it stands to reason that migraine may be caused in many ways. Our understanding of who migraine affects and how it creates such malaise has evolved since the dawn of thought. If we look through the history, we will be able to build a picture of what kind of person was thought to suffer, and what it was about what they did that brought on such malaise.

Given that we have evidence that migraine was being experienced by humans millennia ago, you might think that we have a rich resource by which to work out what it is that makes us so unfortunate as to have our lives touched by this spectre. The demons of ancient times seemed to be indiscriminate; there was no thought given to the individual characteristics of those who were struck down by migraine. By contrast, literature dating from the 19th century, which is often dismissed or ignored by modern scientific and clinical literature, was prolific in its descriptions of the migraine attack, providing a vividness that there seems to be no space to provide nowadays. No one wants to reinvent the wheel, but we should also not ignore what that wheel looks like.

Ancient thought to modern times

In the past, there have been many theories about the causes of migraine and descriptions of the symptoms in literature. For example, the causes outlined by Hippocrates,[1] the first to describe the migraine aura around 400 BCE, took two forms, the first of which was 'humoral'. The humours in Hippocrates' theory were the four bodily fluids: blood, phlegm, yellow bile and black bile, all of which needed to be kept in balance for good health. Illness was caused when these fluids became out of balance, sometimes requiring the reduction in the body of a humour through bloodletting or purging.

Several hundred years later, in the 1st century CE, the celebrated Greek physician Aretæus of Cappadocia put forward an alternative theory: 'The cause of these symptoms is coldness with dryness.' Sorted. So all we need to do to avoid migraine is stay warm and wet! If only it were that simple.

In the 6th century CE, Alexander Trallianus turned back to the humours and suggested that migraine may be caused by an excess of the yellow and black bile, collectively called the bilious humours. Anything that caused the movement of yellow and black bile to the stomach would result in tummy upset. Equally, constipation was seen as a preamble to migraine. Treatment was based on remedies that would purge these humours through the action of emetics that make you vomit, laxatives for defecation and bloodletting to, well, let blood.

This humoral theory wasn't totally wrong: bile is indeed released by the liver and the gall bladder to break down fatty foods. However, Trallianus's theory was wrong in that it erroneously categorised those who experienced migraine as those who ate a decadent, high-fat diet. Migraineurs were therefore encouraged to become sparse in their dietary habits, eschewing high-fat and -protein foods such as butter, meat pies, hot buttered toast, ales... To some, this meant they had to deny themselves anything good in their lives. Puritanicals such as the British Quaker John Fothergill of the 18th century, for instance, saw this as both salvation from his lifelong migraine but also validation of his abstinent ways and teachings.

The second cause of migraine was purported by Hippocrates to be 'sympathetic' in nature. This idea grew as humoral theory took hold in 400 BCE but instead of it being related to bodily fluids, it centred on a particular organ of the body, such as the stomach, the bowel or the uterus. From here, there would be some form of unconscious communication throughout the body, spreading the malaise. The Greeks called it 'sympathy' (the root of which can mean either 'feeling' or 'disease') and the Romans called it 'consensus' (an 'agreement of the senses').

The interesting thing about this theory[2] is that, early though it was, it connected the head, or at least the consequences that were found there, to something that happened in the body. This went against the grain of the prevailing common philosophy, which itself has had a lasting legacy. Not only did Aristotle, shortly after Hippocrates' time, argue cogently (yet erroneously) that there was no way the brain had anything to do with the mind, but it also still wasn't accepted even as late as the 17th century that mind and body could be linked. Instead, dualism was the flavour of the day – the philosophical position supported by the Frenchman René Descartes in the early 1600s that our behaviour is controlled by two entities: the mind (and it was still up in the air whether or not this had anything to do with the brain) and the body.

Based on the sympathetic theory, many of the symptoms of migraine, such as nausea or disturbed appetite that was often coincident with menstruation, could be explained. English physician Thomas Willis, who was active in the mid-1600s, advanced our understanding by marrying keen clinical observation with detailed anatomical investigation.[3] The language with which Thomas Willis described the migraineous episode is at once descriptive, metaphorical and gripping. Speaking of one of his patients ('a most noble Lady'), who was 'extremely punished with this Disease'; he described her 'Distemper' (at this time taken to mean 'bad temper') as 'having pitched its tents near the confines of the Brain' and 'had so long besieged its regal tower, yet it had not taken it; for the sick Lady ... found the chief faculties of her soul sound enough.' If I were to write a scientific paper with this kind of language today, I'd be butt-bounced before it even went to review; it would never be allowed. What a loss in the name of progress. Thomas had, however, correctly identified that even though a person could be completely incapacitated by a migraine, they are fundamentally non-fatal.

We find ourselves now dealing with theories that might point to the migraine's cause. Is it a psychological issue? Is it something to do with a lack of constitutional strength? Is it behavioural, maybe because you like a bacon butty?

Were you born that way? Thomas, for once, put it very succinctly and yet didn't answer the question either...

'...An evil or weak constitution of the parts ... sometimes innate and hereditary ... an irritation in some distant member or viscera ... changes of season atmospheric states, the great aspects of the sun and moon, violent passions and errors in diet.'

That pretty much covers everything, doesn't it, as well as conflating predisposing and behavioural conditions. Let's break this down a bit.

Is it me?

What does the migrainous constitution look like? It's not like we can identify somebody who is prone to migraine walking down the street, although we might spot somebody if they were in the throes of one. Here, we rely on observational correlations. Which of the following clinical characteristics is true?

1 Migraine is much more prevalent in people under 1.6m (5ft 3in) tall.
2 A luxuriant head of hair indicates a migraineur.
3 Migraine is more widespread in women.
4 If you have an inverted nipple, chances are you get migraine.
5 Migraine is commonly seen in red-headed women.

True or not, all have been reported in the scientific literature. This illuminates the age-old problem we have in academic enquiry: the difference between correlation and causation. *Correlating* the greater prevalence of migraine among the bountiful of follicle does not mean that good hair growth *causes* it. On the other hand, we do know that women suffer more from migraine than men, but this is because of the hormonal link, which we will discuss later; there is a *cause* here related to female physiology.

Grace Touraine and George Draper, psychiatrists from New York, sought to define a classic migraine type in their writing in 1934 and settled on a person with some bulbous features about their skull, high intelligence but an unsettled emotional make-up. The hormone link gave the (mostly male) clinicians of the 1900s licence to restrict their comments, outside of their own experiences with migraine of course, almost exclusively to the female of the species and in particular with respect to their form and purported intellect. In 1959, American physician Walter Alvarez wrote about 'Some Characteristics of the Migrainous Woman' observing that such women dressed their small, trim bodies with firm breasts well, were eager of mind and were socially very attractive. They also seemed to age well. Who wouldn't want to suffer from migraine if it meant we got to be the kind of woman Walter saw in his clinic?

Discussion of the psychological underpinnings was similarly conflated between observational correlations and causal attribution. Herman Selinsky, another American physician, writing in 1939, accepted that the headache of migraine was related to vascular changes, but he wanted to understand common psychological factors in his group of 200 migraine patients (with a ratio of four females to every male in the sample) with a view to developing a therapy in this domain. Herman argued that the migraine episode could be seen as a mechanism of escape for the patient from a bad situation, that it could be used to evoke sympathy and not the anger that the situation that brought about the migraine might more appropriately deserve. In his observations, Herman thought that the harassed housewife was very prone to migraine, particularly if they had intellectual leanings that could not be expressed through 'the bearing and raising of children under adverse economic conditions, and the constant drudgery of housework'. They just had no ethical, moral or social way to release the pressure.

This might have made sense in its time but doesn't really get us to the real *cause* of migraine, rather it tries to explain the *function* of migraine – what it was for, what it served to do. The best we can deduce from this kind of theory is that these situations may be coincident with migraine, but the population statistics of the time don't stand up to the argument that every harassed housewife got migraine. What is it about the ones who do that made their stress manifest in this way? And was stress the only cause? The people whom Grace Touraine, George Draper, Herman Selinsky and others met in the 1930s tended to be:

> '....often of an intellectual type with a tendency to worry, rigidity of attitude, driving ambition, exaggerated sense of responsibility, marked sensitiveness to critics and meticulous attitude towards work or responsibility. Furthermore in women, there is usually impairment of ability to achieve sexual gratification.'[4]

In this framework, the migraine was seen as a psycho-physiological outcome and such leaps of logic made it difficult to define the underlying cause, and sometimes masked it. Having inverted nipples or red hair doesn't *cause* migraine. Is there some unifying factor that can tie this together with a possible propensity for high intellect and the sexual dysfunction? Is it possible to separate clinical observations from their time and the social pressures that existed within it? Could it really be true that only intelligent people experienced migraine?

It took until 1971 and William Estlin Water's epidemiological studies to debunk this myth. (The word epidemiology comes from the Greek *epidemia*, meaning the prevalence of disease. Epidemiological studies look at the incidence, spread and control of diseases and health disorders.) In his preferred sample, the population of South Wales, he didn't find any evidence that those who suffered from migraine were more intelligent than those who didn't, but he did see a hint that those who were of higher social standing *and* more intelligent were *more likely to consult a doctor*. After all, not everybody would have had access to a doctor before the 1950s, certainly in the UK, and so this skewed the view of John Fothergill and others throughout history that migraine only existed in the decadently fed, posh and clever domain. It turns out, migraine does not respect these factors at all.

The point of peas

A more biological approach is required and our eye will first fall on heritability as predicted by Thomas Willis back in 1654. The prevalence of traits, and of course illness, in families was noted in ancient times but it wasn't until the late 19th century that Gregor Mendel formalised the science of what we now know as the field of genetics (from the Greek *genesis*, meaning 'origin').

Gregor was an Augustinian Friar who lived in Moravia (now in the Czech Republic), and over the course of seven feverish years, starting in 1856, he noted what happened when he bred and cross-bred pea plants that had different characteristics, such as their height, pea shape and colour, and many others. He realised that there were invisible 'factors' that determined what trait was passed on, and in what proportion in the offspring. For example, when a green pea plant was crossed with a yellow pea plant, only yellow pea plants resulted in the first generation. This is an example of a 'dominant trait': yellow always wins. But curiously, in the next generation, there are three yellow to one green pea plant, and so the green isn't lost completely, it's a trait that is lurking in the background. Gregor called this a 'recessive trait'. He didn't know what these invisible factors were, the 'units of inheritance' as he called them.

He published his results in 1866, which was very lucky because then it was in the public domain. If he hadn't published, the knowledge would have been lost since all of Gregor's papers were burned on his death in 1884 to end a tax dispute he had had with the local government in his capacity as abbot of the monastery.[5]

These units of inheritance, or 'genes' as we now know them, were more clearly defined 30 years later when Mendel's work was rediscovered. Sitting on the chromosomes, or genetic material in every nucleus of every cell, the genes determine what proteins are made. These proteins are the building blocks of every material that can be found in our body. As we touched on in Chapter 5, environment also has a role to play in this. For instance, if you have two genetically identical plants and you raise one with ample water and the other without, one will grow much taller than the other.

Another example is Dolly, the first cloned sheep. Born in July 1996, Dolly looked different to the ewe that donated the original cell containing the genetic material. Keith Campbell, Ian Wilmut and their team at the Roslin Institute in Scotland tried using lots of different body cells with their full complement of 46 chromosomes but they went with the udder one in the end. (See what I did there...) It was because this cell originally came from a mammary gland that the cloned sheep was given the name Dolly...[6]

Dolly died when she was just over six-and-a-half years old, having had six lambs of her own in the regular way (Bonnie, twins Sally and Rosie, and triplets Lucy, Darcy and Cotton). That's a bit of a short life for a Finn Dorset sheep, which is what she was; we might expect them to live until 11 or 12 years old. That said, it's fair to think that because Dolly's genetic, or first, 'mum' – a white-faced Finn Dorset – was six years old when she 'donated' her mammary cell that actually Dolly was six years old on the day she was born; there are a couple of age-related characteristics of her DNA that support this. However, Keith and Ian think that the balance of evidence falls elsewhere. Dolly had arthritis from the age of four, a condition that is age-related for sure, and unusual for a four-year-old sheep, but what killed her was a type of lung cancer called pulmonary adenocarcinoma. This was caused by a bug called Jaagsiekte[7] sheep retrovirus, which is quite common in sheep, particularly those kept indoors – as Dolly was for her own security. A retrovirus is a nasty bug because it gets into your cell nucleus and changes the DNA, replicating itself as the cell divides. Apparently, other sheep in her flock died of the same thing, as it is contagious.

Dolly's 'mum' was the ewe that had donated the egg cell. All of the genetic material of that cell was removed; because it was a sex cell, it would only have contained 23 chromosomes (*see* p. 94). And because it was a sex cell, it was the type of cell (called a stem cell) that is built to divide in the unlimited way necessary to create all the cells required to build a body and everything inside it. So, the DNA of Dolly's genetic 'mum' was put into an egg cell from Dolly's ovum 'mum' and the whole kit and caboodle was implanted into the uterus of Dolly's birth-giving, or third, 'mum'. Both the ovum 'mum' and the birth-giving 'mum' were Scottish Blackface sheep. When Dolly was born, the only lamb out of 277 attempts, she was a white-faced Finn Dorset, which provided evidence that it is the *genetic material* that determines breed. And yet the environment she lived in – a pampered indoor sheep palace, totally different to the living conditions of any of her mums – meant that she displayed various differences in how those genes were expressed.

Subfields of genetics

This interaction of environment with genetics is a subfield called 'population genetics' and can be an interesting way to view heritability of traits and particularly disease across evolution.

Epigenetics, on the other hand, looks at how genes and their activity might be altered, but without messing around with the DNA (as the retrovirus does) that codes for a particular protein. These factors sit on top of the heritable traits that Gregor Mendel identified and can be passed on down to offspring as well.

The study of whether we inherit migraine came a little bit late to the game. It made sense to anybody who thought about it that migraine is a family trait – it is incredibly common to find multiple people in one family who complain of it. The mechanism of this was unclear though. In the 1960s and 1970s various theories abounded: that it was linked to a recessive gene, or a dominant gene, or lots of genes, or (my favourite) that there wasn't a clear genetic picture at all. The problem was, all of these studies relied on self-report of family trees of pain, and of course such a process is fraught with error due to misdiagnosis of other family members' malaise and also a bias that existed because nobody wanted to be left out.

William Waters, who worked for the Medical Research Council's epidemiology unit in South Wales, sought to separate all of these biases. He concluded, in 1971, that genetically determined heritability wasn't as big a deal as those before him believed. For him, environment was a much bigger factor; you weren't born with migraine, you acquired it somehow.

One gene to rule the world?

Perhaps again we need to turn to a finer-grained biological study. With all of our advances in our knowledge of genetics, mapping the genome, working out what specific genes do and playing about with their activity, we should have linked 'the migraine' to a specific 'migraine gene' by now, right? Well, instead of there being one gene to rule the migraine world, science has identified a number of candidate genes, changes to each of which raises the risk of migraine. Many of these studies have been done with people who experience migraine with a clearly defined aura for reasons of clearer diagnosis of the migraine headache (not to be confused with any other type). This means that there is the possibility that migraine without aura has a different genetic profile, but as we saw in the previous chapter, the same brain changes may be going on in somebody without aura, it's just that they don't experience them.

We know with some certainty that there is a particular form of migraine called hemiplegic migraine that is passed down through families. Patients experience extreme muscle weakness or pins and needles down half of their face or head or even their body (hence hemiplegia from the original Greek: *hemi* or 'half', *plege* or 'stroke, plague or wound') that can actually border on or tip into paralysis, similar to symptoms of a stroke. However scary, the effects are temporary.

Hemiplegic, or familial, migraine is linked to an autosomal (not linked to the sex chromosomes and so both the mother and father can carry it) dominant gene, meaning that you only need one parent to have the altered gene to pass it on. Even though you might have the gene, though, it isn't necessarily expressed; in some cases no effects are seen at all. We still need to find out why this is so. What are the environmental triggers that turn this gene on? Are they linked to the regular migraine triggers we know about and will talk about shortly? There is a serious game of 'join the dots' to be done here.

When I was starting university, genetics research was the great hope both for understanding humanity and treating the diseases that affected them. Spotting genes that were responsible for cancer, neurological diseases or heart failure, for example, became a boon to the prediction of disease onset opening up the possibility that we could mitigate them somehow. The Human Genome Project was a Herculean international effort to map all of the genes that are found in the human body. It only started in October 1990 but a mere 13 years later, two years ahead of schedule and under budget, the entire human genetic code was elucidated. It's amazing what we can do when we work together.

Up until now, for the most part genetic studies have focused on candidate genes that often were proposed as possibilities due to the coincidence of migraine with other disorders such as epilepsy, for example. Indeed, four candidates have been proposed to explain this shared genetic basis:

1 CACNA1A on chromosome 19 (makes calcium channels)
2 ATP1A2 on chromosome 1 (makes the sodium/potassium pump)
3 SCN1A on chromosome 2 (makes sodium channels)
4 PRRT2 on chromosome 16 (involved in neuro-transmitter release at the synaptic cleft)

All of these are involved in the release of neurotransmitters and/or the balance of ions between the inside of the nerve cell and outside, the importance of which we saw in the previous chapter. If these abnormal genes are not creating the correct proteins, it will lead to problems with the excitability of these cells and how the signal is passed on from one to the next. As we know, these are problems in various degrees in both epilepsy and migraine.

By spotting these genes and following their inheritance down family trees, coupled with how the condition is manifested in these individuals, we can eventually get some kind of handle on the mechanism of how each altered gene leads to behavioural effects we can actually see. If we can understand the role and the power of these genes, then we can work to normalise them. We're not quite there yet, but in theory we can create a normal gene in the lab and change the patient's DNA so that it will forevermore express the normal gene as opposed to the altered one. This can be done using the trickster retroviruses to ferry the correct form of the gene into the cells of body, like the scorpion crossing the river on the back of a frog.

This so-called 'candidate gene' approach has a couple of methodological drawbacks, however. It is incredibly time-consuming because families expressing the altered gene and an associated condition have to be identified and followed, often over generations. Also, while precise for the families it follows, it is not holistic. There may be other genes outside of the candidate chosen that are just as important, that we may miss or, worse, what you are looking at may just have been found by chance and doesn't generalise to other people at all. The sample size is typically very small and the environmental influence is varied to the point where it is difficult to truly know what's going on. Lastly, while candidate genes are identified and followed, it is rare to have each of them followed in the same familial study to look at interactions between their actions.[8]

Another way to define the genetic basis of a disease is to carry out genome-wide association studies (GWAS). Instead of focusing on one or a few genes at a time, looking for problems, we can now mix what we know about the genome with population genetics. What's interesting about this approach is that it doesn't start with a hypothesis – a theory that you are looking to either prove or disprove. The candidate gene approach does this: you might start off by saying 'I think the PRRT2 gene is involved in migraine. Can I prove this?' as opposed to the GWAS, which would merely ask a question like 'what are the genes associated with migraine?' Everything gets reported in this latter case – both the associated genes and the unassociated ones – whereas in the candidate gene approach, only when a hypothesis is proved does publication usually result. This is why I am such a fan of a question-led approach; anything can happen, nothing is off the table, and it is up to you as a scientist to design a good experiment and interpret the results in some kind of intelligent framework based on what we already know, or one that looks beyond to how we might understand something in the future.

It turns out that there are more than 40 genes that can be implicated in migraine. The inheritance of these genes is much higher in hemiplegic migraine than in other forms, and also seems to be higher in those reporting migraine with aura as opposed to without. Three of the four candidate genes for hemiplegic migraine have been confirmed using GWAS, with PRRT2 losing its credibility as a driving factor in the process. Interestingly, even outside of this most clearly hereditable form of migraine, there is a genetic basis for specific clinical features of other migraine that can be passed down. A strong family history of migraine incidence is associated with a lower age of onset, more frequent migraine episodes and migraine with aura. GWAS studies looking at populations of people who experience migraine without aura also shows robust genetic associations, but there are subtle differences with aura populations probably leading to their threshold of aura consciousness being different. Overall, these two migraine subtypes are more alike than different.

What's the point?

So, migraine is in our genome, with at least one form being distinctly genetically heritable (remember, familial heritability takes the environment into account also). But this makes no sense. Migraine is a figurative pain in the ass and a literal pain almost everywhere else. What use is it to us as human beings in the 21st century?

The human body is adept at letting redundant features go throughout the course of evolution. We have no use for the appendix any more, since we no longer have the kind of diet it was useful for, since it helped us digest the foods we no longer eat so much of. We also have little use for wisdom teeth, those huge brutes that break through our gums in our teenage years (as if we didn't have enough going on), again because our diet has changed. 'OK,' evolution said, 'I take your point'; both appendices and wisdom teeth are being selected out of the genome as we speak. At least one in 100,000 people are born without an appendix, and they are only spotted because of surgery or scans for something else, they never knew, and so the number could be much higher. Up to 35 per cent of people will never cut wisdom teeth.

Other adaptations include the fact that kids are being born nowadays with better musculature and control over their thumb movements, to deal with the requirements of video games and swiping apps. These are the offspring of the Nintendo generation, who began to adapt to such movements, and because it was advantageous to do so this trait was passed down to the next generation. (I am of the Atari generation; I'm not sure any good came from that aside from a love of Pong.)

The bottom line of evolution is this: adaptations (either accidental ones like mutations, or experiential ones) that help our species survive and make life easier and/or more efficient will eventually be passed down. Altered genes or mutations that are not helpful will not. So why do we still have migraine?

We might make the same argument for depression, the most common affective mood disorder out there. Our moods are complex but are generally driven by two main aspects of thinking behaviour; we all use varying levels of a problem-solving approach and a more reflective brooding approach. A greater propensity to the brooding approach is coincident with the onset of depressive symptoms. Given the genetic basis of personality type and thinking style, one might think that given the risk of a brooding style to the onset of depression we should have selected that out of our genome already, because there is nothing helpful about depression, right? Wrong. I recently supervised a PhD student called Yan Birch, who was puzzled by this from his undergrad days. He did a series of experiments that showed that a brooding, thinking style was *really* important for certain thinking tasks. Sure, a more problem-solving approach was important in some other tasks, but brooding allows us to bring extra neural resources to the table, allowing us to dwell on problems we find it hard to break down.

Of course, at some point, this can become maladaptive – we use up a lot of our neurotransmitters like serotonin in the process of the work our brain is doing and if we are not replenishing them as we go through our behaviours and interactions with others then we can fall into an emotional hole with increasingly negative thoughts. However, the critical point is that we *need* this kind of thinking to solve problems, so it would be detrimental to us to have selected our ability to do it out of our genome.

So, is there any evidence that we *need* migraine? For example, it could be that migraine has a beneficial side effect – as is the case with the mutation that causes sickle cell anaemia, which also gives you protection from malaria – although it appears that there's nothing so striking going on. We could also look at this from a behavioural evolutionary perspective, as Herman Selinsky did, back in New York in the 1930s, in effect saying that migraine is required to save the harassed housewife. (A pretty extreme measure I would have thought, even in 1939.) However, his theory comes from too high up in the behavioural tree for me to be happy for it to explain why migraine exists. The vasodilation that happens after the constriction in the migraine pathway could be seen as protective and this causes at least part of the headache, but the migraine experience is so much more. Why are our neurons going bananas in the first place? What's the value of that?

The crimes of fashion against humanity

We have some tantalising evidence – and the first factor lies in the visual system. People who experience migraine have a much more excitable visual cortex than others.

If other parts of the brain weren't involved in processing the visual picture and we just had this area, called V1, we would see the world as a group of lines of every orientation there is. This is because the neurons that are found here respond only to lines, with each cell only firing off an action potential if there is a line of the right orientation appearing in exactly the place in space that neuron is tuned to. You have millions of these neurons, and they all add together successively over the rest of the visual system (with such imaginative names as V2, V3, V4 and V5) to build up the picture and detect edges and movement and overall contrast.

The role of V1 is straightforward. We test this in the lab by giving people very simple visual search tasks to do. For example, you might have to pick out a / from a load of \ forms for a really low-level task that would just occupy V1, or you might have to find a particular car from other pictures of cars, which would require higher-level processing. Back in 1995, Shirley Wray and her colleagues from Harvard showed that migraineurs, who rather crucially were not experiencing a headache at the time, were much faster than control people at the V1 task, but that both groups were as fast as each other at the higher-level task. In the early 2000s, Ed Chronicle from the University of Lancaster and his team showed that this advantage was linked to hyperexcitability of V1, which is similar in those who experience aura and those who don't. This not only explains the extreme photophobia migraineurs experience during the headache but it also seems that even outside of the migraine episode these neurons are on a hair trigger for activation.

Opticians are already well aware of how much more sensitive a migraineur's peripheral vision is. We can prove this in the lab by sending magnetic pulses into your brain to generate the phosphenes or spots of light we talked about in the previous chapter. It takes much less stimulation to generate a phosphene in somebody who gets migraine than other people. There are lots of things that affect the reactivity of your brain to stimulation like this (as I know after spending a gazillion hours in the lab, many stimulating myself for scientific kicks [this sounds bad, the insertion of the word 'scientific' didn't help at all]) but the lower threshold for migraineurs is there no matter what. In addition to behavioural tests (e.g. the visual search one described above) and transcranial magnetic stimulation, you can also detect this difference using a visceral response. Flash up a picture of an Indian rug featuring lines going in lots of different directions and the response from your audience at the regional Migraine Society meeting will tell you all you need to know. In addition to not making any friends, I learned some new curse words from that audience. Tough crowd.

This can happen much closer to home and is often something people don't think about. Venetian blinds? Invention of the devil. If you have an excitable visual cortex, just imagine the torture you are putting it through if you are surrounded by venetian blinds in your house, activating all of the neurons selective for horizontal lines all at once. These bladed blinds were actually invented in Persia, but were introduced to Europe by the Venetians in 1760. The French resisted the credit belonging to Venice though and still call them Persian blinds (Les Persiennes). As a migraine sufferer myself, I have a different (but impolite) name for them; in fact, if hell is a place, it is shaded by venetian blinds. By the end of the 19th century they were everywhere, in homes, churches and courthouses, even being present to witness the signing of the American Declaration of Independence in 1774. Immortalised in art by American Impressionist Edmund Charles Tarbell, his picture, descriptively named 'The Venetian Blind' (1898) depicts the back of a scantily clad woman in a recumbent pose in front of a venetian blind. I'm not surprised; she probably had a killer migraine. Perhaps actually the woman was Venetian and she was blinded by the light in her malaised state. Or perhaps I am reading too much into it...

Yet we are surrounded by lines so much so in fact that we really don't notice them most of the time. But sometimes, they will rankle. About a year ago I had a really bad migraine that I just couldn't seem to shift – it kept coming back over the course of two weeks. I had my eyes tested. I even went to the dentist to make sure I didn't have anything going on in my teeth. It turned out that my wife had been shopping and had taken to wearing lots of stripy tops, some of them with tightly packed black-and-white lines. Well, you may as well have given me arsenic. I forbade her to wear them in my presence again and my headache went away. I am used to sharing meetings with men in stripy shirts but I am not contractually obliged to give them the whole of my visual attention, and so that doesn't affect me so much. Marriage, on the other hand, is different.[9]

It's not just lines that the hyperactive visual cortex is sensitive to; it can also be flashing lights and strip fluorescent lights that are slightly out of phase with each other. These are commonly found in clothing stores – another reason why I don't like to shop. Migraineurs can detect a much more subtle flicker in strip lighting than the rest of the population.

The hyperactive visual cortex can be linked to abnormal neurotransmitter balance, in particular a lack of inhibitory control. And the migraine features, namely the wave of excitability that starts off the cortical spreading depolarisation followed by the depression, are triggered by a certain spatial frequency, or how close together the lines are. That's why not all patterns of lines around us set it off, and it's fair to say that every migraineur might have a different spatial frequency that triggers them. Activate every single V1 neuron by presenting lines of every orientation packed together in a neat rectangle, though, and you will trigger all sufferers.

But back to evolution. The value of having a very sensitive primary visual cortex lies in your ability to see very small contrasts and other differences in the visual scene. This will have been of value in our hunter-gatherer past, for picking out movement of potential predators or prey in tall grass or trees. Also, because your V1 is very sensitive, you will be able to maximise the signals coming from your retina, making your vision more acute in dim light. By this view, migraineurs are evolutionarily *more advanced*. Said no migraineur, ever.

Other badges in biology

In other news, there is a lesser incidence of alcoholism in people who experience migraine, but this may be due to the individual protecting themselves from alcohol-induced headache and not really show an evolutionary advantage at all.

On the other hand, Knut Hagen followed 70,000 people in Norway over the course of 10 years and found that those with a diagnosis of Type 1 diabetes had a much lower incidence of migraine. There may be a genetic link here, or a behavioural one in that Type 1 diabetics tend to be more controlled about what they eat. In this study, no link was found between Type 2 diabetes and migraine but a French 10-year study did find that women were up to 30 per cent less likely to develop Type 2 diabetes if they got migraines. Although these migraines were self-reported and therefore sensitive to misdiagnoses, this number is too high to ignore; migraine seems to be protective against developing Type 2 diabetes. Again, this might be because those who suffer from headaches are much more careful around foods thought to be migraine triggers, thus perhaps having healthier eating habits, and so lessening the chance of developing diabetes. Or perhaps if we turn this on its head, there may be something about elevated blood sugar that stops headaches from happening and the chocolate (and carbs) that we crave in the prodrome phase may be self-medication with sugar and is not particularly serotonin-related after all.

Alternatively, there may be a link with proteins that may be found in abundance in migraine but not diabetes. One such candidate is calcitonin gene-related peptide (CGRP). This is released in great quantities as part of the cortical spreading depression we came across in the last chapter, but is actually produced to a lesser degree following the onset of diabetes. It's a protein that is important in the inflammatory response in the tissues of the body and part of this is the proper regulation of fuel to the brain and other tissues of the body. This may be the link between migraine and diabetes. Too much CRGP leads to pain, too little leads to high blood sugar. And one precludes the other.

Knowing this means we can target CRGP as a new treatment for migraine. If we block the receptors on which CRGP works, we can cut off the inflammatory response and so the pain signals. This is the culmination of work Peter Goadsby from UCL and his colleagues have been doing since the early 1990s. Called Erenumab, it is injected below the skin and improved migraine incidence in 30 per cent of patients in the test group, but only 14 per cent in the control group. The actual improvement seen over the placebo effect is a 16 per cent decrease in incidence. It offers another mode of treatment for those in whom acute treatment such as sumatriptan doesn't work. (You might remember sumatriptan as being a good treatment for cluster headache. It is a serotonin agonist acting just like serotonin in the brain and also constricts the vasodilation that causes the pain in migraine.)

We've talked before about how we might start to try to self-medicate with chocolate and sex to boost our serotonin levels and so if not head off (sorry) a headache at least treat ourselves in some other way. But it turns out that we do this already, all of the time! Tim Houle looked at sexual desirability scores in a sample of Chicagoans who suffered from either tension headache or migraine. He found that men were 24 per cent more interested in sex than women (not hugely surprising) but that women who experience migraine are right up there with the average man for sexual desire. Overall, migraineurs desired sex 20 per cent more than those who suffered from tension headache. Serotonin is therefore a big factor in the migraine mix (but not tension headache), explaining why taking a serotonin mimic works for some migraineurs, as well as people with cluster headache.

In fact, migraineurs tend to have *lower* serotonin levels than the rest of the population; genome-wide association studies reveal that migraine shares the same genetic variant risks as depression. There is a higher co-incidence of migraine with depression and the underlying pathway, at least in part, relates to this serotonin imbalance. Selective serotonin-reuptake inhibitors that make serotonin hang around in the synapse for longer may help raise and stabilise serotonin levels in migraine as they do in depression. However, behavioural mechanisms such as social connectedness, fun, satisfaction and love all work to sustain them over time.

The menstrual migraine

For women, there is a further clear hormonal pathway to trigger migraine. Three times more women than men suffer from migraine and of these women, 70 per cent experience menstrual migraine. It's the fluctuation of hormones that is the culprit here. The menstrual cycle is roughly 28 days long and has four distinct but overlapping phases. Day one is counted as the first day of menstruation when all hormones are at their lowest levels. The follicular phase starts on the first day of your period and lasts right up to ovulation. In this phase, the hypothalamus (the puppet master of the endocrine system) kicks the pituitary gland into gear to release follicle-stimulating hormone (FSH), which does exactly what it says. About 20 follicles, or cyst-like nodules, each carrying an immature ovum or egg, form on the surface of the ovary. The developing follicles release oestrogen to coincide with the end of menstruation, which encourages a thickening of the lining of the uterus in preparation for receipt of a mature egg. The hypothalamus detects the increase in oestrogen and in reply it prompts the pituitary to release luteinising hormone (LH) – from the Latin *luteum* for 'egg yolk' – and another burst of FSH. The levels of all three – oestrogen, LH and FSH – peak just before ovulation, when a mature egg[10] bursts out of one of the follicles and is swept up by the oviduct (or Fallopian tube, named after Gabriello Fallopio, the Italian anatomist who described them in the 16th century), which transports the egg to the uterus.

While oestrogen, LH and FSH levels are falling following ovulation, the burst follicle gradually seals itself off, transforming into a structure called the corpus luteum. The corpus luteum releases progesterone and a little bit of oestrogen. Both of these maintain the thickened lining of the uterus, waiting to see if a fertilised egg will implant in its folds. If it does, then the corpus luteum sticks around and keeps up the release of progesterone and oestrogen. But if not, it just withers away by day 12, just like the unused follicles at ovulation do. Progesterone and oestrogen are no longer released by the dead corpus luteum and so concentrations fall, meaning the lining of the uterus falls away by day 28, starting the menstrual cycle all over again. Menstrual migraines are mostly linked to the last few days or the first few days of the menstrual cycle, a time when hormone levels are fluctuating from high to low and back again.

More evidence that fluctuating oestrogen levels are implicated in the incidence of migraine comes from Simone Ferrero, a gynaecologist from the University of Genoa. She and her team found that women with endometriosis are more than twice as likely to suffer migraine as women without it. Endometriosis is when the lining of the uterus, the endometrium, forms outside of the uterus itself and sticks to organs and tissues in the abdominal cavity; it can be incredibly painful and debilitating and a greater propensity for migraine is all the poor patient needs. Some 13.5 per cent of the women in the endometriosis group experienced migraine with aura, in comparison with 1.2 per cent of the control group who did not have endometriosis.

Coupled with the fact that endometriosis presents with high oestrogen levels, it may be that there is a causal link between oestrogens and cortical spreading depolarisation and the threshold by which individuals are conscious of its perceptual effects. Low oestrogen seems to be linked to migraine without aura and so the role of oestrogen may lie in how we actually experience the aura. Oestrogens can certainly play with neuronal excitability in lots of ways, and they interact with the blood vessels of the brain. In the case of endometriosis, though, there are added factors causing pain, such as the release of prostaglandins and nitric oxide, which are both part of the inflammatory response and direct stimulators of the trigeminal nerve.

There is some evidence that migraine is related to lower levels of gonadal hormones such as oestrogen, progesterone and testosterone in both men and women, but of course, these have a more cyclical role to play in women, increasing the prevalence of their effect. Since all of these hormones are ultimately controlled by the hypothalamus, and if we put this together with the hypothalamic symptoms of the prodrome phase we discovered in Chapter 6, there is of course the chance that hypothalamic dysfunction or, more specifically in this case, underactivity of the hypothalamic–pituitary–gonadal axis could be the root of all of this evil.

The use of external hormones might ease symptoms here as they work to stabilise the hormone concentrations. Because they stop the fluctuation of hormones necessary for the normal conditions whereby an egg is released by setting oestrogen and progesterone to higher-than-normal levels, it removes the possibility of conception. You might know these drugs better as oral contraceptives. The initial dose of oestrogen might lead to migraine to start with (due to the link of high oestrogen with migraine aura) but this tends to stabilise over time.

As we know, the fluctuation of oestrogen from low to high and back again causes various psychoactive effects; it can affect our mood and even our cognitive function. German psychologist Markus Hausmann and his team have investigated various cognitive tasks across the menstrual cycle and have concluded that these changes in hormonal concentration affect the brain such that more of the brain gets involved and functions that would usually require only one side of the brain now include both. Remember Ed Chronicle's view that the hyperactivity in visual cortex in migraine is due to a lack of normal inhibition between the two hemispheres? Put this together with how hormones change the balance of activity across the hemispheres and we begin to get a sense of why our hormonal milieu might set the scene for the migraine episode. Markus has essentially found that these hormone-induced changes in brain activity in women do mean that they find it hard to engage the spatial perception required to parallel park. But don't get carried away, fellas, the effect is very limited to a specific and relatively small window in the menstrual cycle. Quit your generalising.

The heart of the matter

There is another, perhaps surprising bodily function that may cause migraine, and it lies in your heart. This is a pretty vital organ, which takes all the deoxygenated blood from your body into its right chambers and redirects it straight to the lungs to become oxygenated again. The left side of the heart gathers all of this lovely oxygenated blood and redirects it around your body. It's a pump, and it can beat faster or slower depending on the demands of your body for blood to various areas, and that's governed by the autonomic system.

Before you were born and you were in utero, even though your lungs were developing, you didn't breathe through them (if you did, you would have got a lungful of amniotic fluid and that wouldn't be good). So even though your circulatory system was developing to prepare you to breathe normally when you were born, there wasn't really any point in the blood being diverted to the lungs because there was no oxygen there to collect. You got all your oxygen through the umbilical cord from the placenta; this is where the transfer of oxygen occurs, instead of the lungs. This problem is taken care of quite easily in the developing foetus by having an open passage between the top chambers (called the atria) of the heart, which are usually separated by an impenetrable wall called the septum. Blood comes in from the body in the regular way on the right side but then instead of being redirected to the lungs, it passes through the septum of the atria using a gap called the foramen ovale (literally an oval hole). The left side of the heart then redistributes this blood around the foetal body.

After birth, the foramen ovale is sealed shut in 75–80 per cent of people. But in some people it is left open or 'patent', leading to the condition's name: patent foramen ovale. It can be left completely open, requiring surgery at birth, or it can be incompletely closed, by a flap of tissue in the atrial septum. This doesn't always cause symptoms and you might never know that it's there, but when pressure is created in the chest by coughing or sneezing the flap can open. This means that at that moment, blood can flow in either direction between the right and left atria. The problem isn't so much to do with oxygenated or deoxygenated blood ending up in the wrong place if the flap only opens rarely. The issue for the brain's purposes is what else the blood contains. If blood passes from the right atrium to the left atrium and is distributed around the body, then it means it hasn't passed through the lungs yet. This is important, because as well as oxygenating the blood the lungs act as an important filtration system for the circulating blood, removing bits of debris, such as small blood clots, for example. Although the kidneys do this too, it is the primary function of the spleen, making it an incredibly important (and my second-favourite) organ in the body, even if it is the first thing to be removed in medical dramas on television.

Essentially, there is a direct route for unfiltered blood to get to the brain. Once there, the cerebrovascular system's arteries (that carry oxygenated blood) branch off into smaller arterioles and tiny capillaries where any of this debris can get stuck, and if it does it stops the blood flow to that part of the brain, directly affecting its activity. In a worst-case scenario, these neurons die due to the lack of oxygen and nutrients, and this is the basis of both transient ischemic attacks (where blood flow in the brain is temporarily blocked) and also its scary big brother, ischemic stroke (where the blockage is longer-lasting and causes brain damage).

You can see how this phenomenon might link to migraine. A small piece of debris blocking a blood vessel in the brain will not only alter the activity there but will also set up rebounds both with respect to compensatory overactivation of the neurons in the brain (setting up the wave of excitation underlying cortical spreading depression) and rebound surrounding inflammation and vasodilation to cope with the ischemic area. However, it took until 2005 to correlate the coincidence of patent foramen ovale with people who experience migraine. Markus Schwerzmann and his team from Bern, Switzerland, compared 93 migraine patients with 93 controls. They found that 47 per cent of the migraine group had a patent foramen ovale in comparison with 17 per cent of controls, and while the control ovales tended to be small, the migraine sufferers were more likely to have mid-sized or large gaps with a right-to-left flow between the atria. None of these people know that they even had this condition – many don't until they suffer a stroke or other medical emergency.

So, now we can look for patent foramen ovale as a possible anatomical cause for migraine. Once this is known, treatment becomes more straightforward. Beta blockers, which interact with the autonomic control of your heart – meaning your heart beats more slowly and with less force – have shown some success. Blood thinners can help, although I always think these are poorly named. The likes of aspirin or warfarin don't actually make your blood thinner or break up clots, but they can stop you forming new ones and slow the growth of the ones you already have. Anti-coagulant is a much more representative moniker.

Warfarin and its uses

Warfarin, which we've been using for more than 60 years, stops the formation of vitamin K-dependant clotting factors in your liver. It was first discovered after herds of cows died in North America and Canada from a bleeding disorder that happened either spontaneously or through nicks and scrapes. In 1930, Lee Rodrick from North Dakota realised that this had to do with an anti-coagulant that was made when sweet clover went bad, and that all the cows who had died had been given mouldy silage made from clover.

Ten years later, Karl Link and his student Harold Campbell from the University of Wisconsin – Madison isolated the chemical that was causing the complete breakdown of the clotting system and called it 4-hydroxy coumarin. Ten years after that, the reality that coumarin could be used as a biological weapon against rats sank in and warfarin was first developed, getting its name as a hybrid of the funders of the work (the Wisconsin Alumni Research Foundation, WARF) and the chemical it comes from (coum-*arin*). By 1954, its medical value to humans was defined, thankfully in much lower doses than are contained in the rat poison. It remains the most widely used anti-coagulant in the world, irrespective of the side effects of bleeding that can occur.

It is, however, possible now to heal the incompletely sealed flap that may be causing all the problems. In 2007, cardiologist Michael Mullen and his team at London's Royal Brompton Hospital developed a bioabsorbable (something that can be absorbed by living tissue) patch that acts as a temporary plug, allowing the body's healing response to cover it over and replace it with normal healthy tissue. This only takes 30 days to do in the body – all it needed was a bridge. It's an improvement on the previous grafting procedure, which often led to inflammation problems, because it was permanently present and seen as a foreign object by the body. The best thing of all is that the patch is carried into a body through a catheter, a flexible tube that wends its way through the vascular system from the groin, where it is inserted. The operator can see where they are going as the catheter also contains a tiny camera that beams back live pictures from inside your body. I'm guessing you can tell how fascinated I am by this. When the catheter gets to the right place in the heart, it deposits the patch and your immune system does the rest!

Why migraine, why now?

The reasons why people get migraine are myriad. So far, we know it can be baked into our biology through genetic factors and that these may (or may not) affect how excitable our visual cortex is, how we produce sex hormones, how many inflammatory proteins like CGRF we have floating around our systems and the anatomical development of our heart. But what about the role of environmental factors like tiredness, stress or diet? Well, these aren't so different to triggers for other headaches. The difference lies in how you and your brain, as a migraineur, react to them.

Migraine is a neurovascular headache. Triggers can affect the neural activity of the brain directly (as stripy lines do) or may have an impact on the vasculature that indirectly affects brain activity, both generating the specific migraine experience. The fact that there is such a thing as a special 'migraineous brain' determines why everybody doesn't get them.

Treat yourself right

We saw in the previous chapter that there has been a tremendous amount of misunderstanding about so-called 'trigger foods'; foods that our hypothalamus encourages us to eat in the prodrome phase don't actually trigger the migraine, it is just our brain yanking our chain. You have an urge to eat chocolate, eat the chocolate! But are we throwing the baby out with the bathwater? Are there some foods or dietary habits that really *can* cause the migraine experience? When I talk to migraineurs, they often mention that missing meals or fasting can invariably lead to a migraine. This stands to reason and is not always restricted to migraine headache; it happens in tension headache, too. This is because vasodilation will occur to maximise the delivery of glucose to the brain if concentrations are low, but of course, as we now know, this will have specific effects in the migraineous brain.

Dana Turner, who works in North Carolina with Tim Houle (who, you might remember, was interested in how interested migraineurs were in having sex) and others, asked 34 migraineurs who experienced at least two headaches a month with headaches present between 4 and 14 days in the month to keep a diary for six weeks. When they looked in detail at the diary days that followed a non-headache day (to reduce any changes in behaviour that might have been induced by the headache) they found that night-time snacking resulted in a 40 per cent drop in the odds of experiencing a headache as opposed to having no food at night. Eating a late dinner resulted in a 21 per cent decrease in the chances of a headache developing with respect to having no food, but the difference here wasn't statistically significance (and so could have equally been due to chance).

The snacking finding was significant though. Putting this finding together with what we know about migraineurs having more inflammation-causing calcitonin gene-related peptide (CGRP) floating around their systems, we might suggest that utilising that CGRP in its fuel regulation role gives it less chance to get involved in its inflammatory activities. This fits well with the protective effect of migraine for diabetes (people who get migraines are much less likely to develop diabetes); high blood sugar might stop headaches, low blood sugar causes them.

I spend a lot of time debunking the chocolate myth with migraineurs, but they will often cite other triggers such as cheese, Chinese food and processed foods. Tyramine is a unifying factor here as it is present in many ripened and aged cheeses such as Camembert and Brie but also soy sauce, miso, cured meats and fish.

Tyramine is a simple neurotransmitter called a monoamine – just like serotonin and dopamine are – that regulates our blood pressure by causing vasoconstriction. Too much of it, or indeed too little of the monoamine oxidase that breaks it down and removes the excess from our bodies (which leads to too much tyramine in our systems) can lead to vascular changes. Given how sensitive our brains are to vascular changes, and migraineous brains in particular, this might explain why these foods cause headaches.

What's more, monoamine oxidase inhibitors (MOIs), which are often prescribed for depression since they stop the breakdown of mood-affecting neurotransmitters such as serotonin and dopamine, will also inhibit the breakdown of excess tyramine. For this reason, eating a meal that's high in tyramine while taking MOIs can lead to serious hypertension (high blood pressure) because of overconstriction of the blood vessels.

The MSG argument

A further link with Chinese food is the presence of monosodium glutamate (MSG), a substance that is found in lots of other cooking and products too, and naturally in mushrooms, seaweed, tomatoes and soy, and also Parmesan cheese, among other things. The additive form was first developed in 1908 by a Japanese chemist called Kikunae Ikeda at Tokyo Imperial University, who was fascinated by the factors that gave his food flavour. He noticed that if kombu, a type of kelp, was added to the broth, it made his soup taste delicious. Some further investigation led him to identify the fifth human taste, umami, and that what those taste receptors are detecting is glutamate, a building block of proteins. As Kikunae pointed out, we have no doubt developed a taste for glutamate because it indicates the presence of vital proteins we should be ingesting to keep us alive.

Glutamate itself doesn't have the umami flavouring but it activates the glutamate receptors in the taste buds in the mouth, which our brain detects as a savoury meaty flavour. In effect, it adds punch to somewhat tasteless dishes. However, it took 100g (4oz) of dried kelp to isolate 1g of glutamate through a very long and convoluted process, so for his next trick, Kikunae set about trying to make this easier for the purposes of home cooking. He needed something with the physical characteristics of salt or sugar to add to stock bases and the like. With this template in mind, he looked for chemicals to buddy up with the glutamate that would be granular and robust to moisture and humidity but be soluble in water. The isolated glutamate by itself looks like little brown crystals and are very powerful; distribution within the bond of another chemical would lower the concentration and make it much easier to work with. Sodium was the ideal candidate and the resultant bond between one molecule of sodium to every glutamate molecule became the salt-like monosodium glutamate. Kikunae knew he'd cracked it and called the new seasoning *Ajinomoto* (味の素) or 'essence of flavour'. It duly went into mass production in 1909 using a more efficient method than the kelp procedure (it now involves wheat and soybeans) and today, the Ajinomoto Company, Inc. employs more than 32,000 people in 35 countries.

MSG is down as a migraine trigger in the current version of International Classification of Headache Disorders. The problem is, the evidence is ropey beyond feedback from migraine sufferers, and the mechanism by which it might cause headaches isn't very clear at all.

The controversy started in 1968 when Robert Ho Man Kwok wrote a short letter to the *New England Journal of Medicine* that was subsequently published. At the time, he was a medical doctor working as a senior research investigator at the National Biomedical Research Foundation in Maryland. He explained that he had regular symptoms following his visits to Chinese restaurants since his arrival in America, experiencing 'numbness in the back of the neck, gradually radiating to both arms and the back, general weakness, and palpitation.' He discounted the high salt content as well as the cooking wine and soy sauce (which was weird, considering the fact that the latter contains both tyramine and glutamate) as triggers, saying he cooked with them at home and they didn't have any effect. He suggested that perhaps it was the monosodium glutamate that is used liberally as seasoning in Chinese restaurants, particularly cuisine from the north of China, and called other doctors to arms in the investigation of this theory. Because he titled his letter 'Chinese Restaurant Syndrome' he not only coined a new pejorative phrase (it was later changed to 'MSG symptom complex') and validated the malaise but he also sparked off years of study and anti-MSG sentiment, forcing Chinese restaurants to advertise that they don't use MSG in their cooking. How did a speculative letter gain such traction in America and across the world so fast?

Published by the Massachusetts Medical Society, the *New England Journal of Medicine* is the oldest and certainly one of the most prestigious medical journals in the world. Its weekly editions contain articles and state-of-play reviews in addition to a letters section that continues to garner lively debate. Its impact factor, which is a measure of how respected it is through how much other people cite its papers, is over 79 points, dwarfing the mere 53 *The Lancet* scores (which is pretty huge too). It's A Big Deal and the journal has historically seen itself as the arbiter of the acceptable – indicating what the scientific community should be interested in. There was a tradition at the time of comic syndrome letters appearing alongside more strait-laced ones in the letters pages of the *New England Journal of Medicine*, often expounding on the phenomenon of common problems with overly scientific, pretentious and clinical language, seemingly just for fun but presumably it floated the boat of the Letters Editor. There was even a letter on Cryogenic Cephalalgia, which all of us reading this book now know as brain freeze, and others on French Vanilla Frostbite, Space Invaders Wrist or Credit-Carditis. This would seem to be how clinicians at the time got their kicks, but in re-reading them, some of them strike me as primers to nascent but possible societal conditions.

In response to Kwok's letter there were many replies, as many completely endorsing the syndrome as there were pooh-poohing it. Then the media, including as respected an outlet as *The New York Times*, got hold of the controversy and the snowball rolled on from there. All argument on the matter soon superseded the role of MSG, appropriating the main thrust of the problem to Chinese food, which was entirely stupid as MSG is found in everything from nature to crisps.

One respondent, Herbert Schaumburg, a pharma-cologist, actually was true to his word and went on to intensively investigate the effect of MSG on human health, designing his tests in collaboration with a neurologist called Robert Byck. They chose to inject MSG in large quantities into 13 people, and this, quite understandably, didn't go so well since MSG is ordinarily ingested and not injected. They did also give MSG orally to participants and noticed symptoms such as burning, facial pressure, chest pain and headache (bear in mind, the original letter never mentioned headache explicitly), although people had vastly different sensitivities to MSG. A big problem with the experiment was that it wasn't blinded (the subjects knew what was being tested), which is a bit like having a biased juror when you are being tried for a crime; in this case, MSG was in the dock. There were also some very strange experiments that involved injecting huge amounts of MSG into baby mice and monkeys, because that's representative of the human experience, not, showing that the mice and monkeys grew up with serious impairments. Well, yes, as glutamate is the most ubiquitous excitatory neurotransmitter in the nervous system, this is hardly surprising.

By 1970, lots of studies were appearing debunking the earlier human studies, but the horse had bolted: it was in the public domain and the public were worried. So much so in fact that in the early 1970s Ralph Nader, a consumer activist and much later a US presidential candidate (in the Bush/Gore/Nader election in 2000), lobbied Congress to ban its use in baby food. This is highly ironic given that glutamate is present in breast milk. Good luck with that one, Ralph.

Since then, loads of studies using placebos have shown that MSG causes no different effects to a placebo substance. But the public were still not convinced. In 1995, the Food and Drug Administration (FDA) in America, decided to put the controversy to bed, asking the Federation of American Societies of Experimental Biology to investigate it thoroughly. It turns out, if you eat six times the normal amount of MSG, on an empty stomach, you might experience something akin to what

Herbert Schaumburg found in his human studies, but the number of people affected by this approach was very small. What's more, the glutamate in MSG does not cross the blood brain barrier and so can't have psychoactive effects or set off cortical spreading depolarisation in migraine, so its effects wouldn't be particular to migraine anyway (which was not mentioned in Ho-Man Kwok's original letter!). So there you go: MSG does not cause migraines, as so many people seem to believe.

Ham-fisted approach

Another, more theoretically sound dietary candidate takes the form of nitrates. Nitrates are naturally occurring chemical compounds that contain nitrogen and oxygen. Found in green leafy vegetables and also carrots and celery (perhaps in slightly lesser concentrations in organic food that has not been exposed to nitrogen-based fertilisers), they are powerful antibacterial agents. It is for this reason that they are added to processed foods such as bacon, sausages, cooked meats – indeed any meat that has been smoked, salted or cured. You might remember that nitric oxide is an important inflammatory substance in the body and it has the power to induce dilation of the blood vessels it is working on. Usually, this is an important mechanism in the cardiovascular system; it keeps blood flow to the heart regular and optimises it for the amount of work it has to do. People with angina, or narrowing of the blood vessels that feed the heart, will often be prescribed a Glyceryl Tri-Nitrate (GTN) spray to be deployed under their tongue when they experience symptoms. The spray serves as a fast way of introducing nitric oxide into the body, causing widespread vasodilation releasing the pressure on the cardiovascular system. However, vasodilation also happens in the cerebrovascular system, often leading to headache following the use of the GTN spray. But we also saw how spiralling levels of nitric oxide induced by muscle hardness can lead to tension headache by tugging on the trigeminal nerve so annoyingly. The ingestion of nitrates, therefore, would seem to be not good for anyone. But is there the chance that migraineurs are more sensitive to ingested nitrates?

For this we need to think about our digestive system, and specifically the mouth. Here, we find lots of substances: saliva, or salivary amylase, an enzyme that is the first to start breaking down the food we ingest; and a whole host of natural flora – bacteria that do the same job. Some of these bacteria work to reduce nitrates into nitrites and then nitric oxide for quick absorption in the body (which is why the GTN spray under the tongue is a clever delivery system).

As part of the Great American Gut Project Cohort in 2016, Antonio Gonzalez, working in Rob Knight's team in the University of California, San Diego, found that there were more bacteria devoted to breaking down nitrates found in foods in the mouth of a migraineur than in those who don't experience migraines. It remains to be seen if this translates into higher concentrations of nitric oxide in the system that may lead to the cerebrovascular effects underlying the typical migraine, or indeed if this difference is causative of migraine, or just an effect. However, it is a rather ingenious way of getting to the root of a problem, and offers another window on why nitrates affect migraineurs in particular. Perhaps this is another protective mechanism of migraine, representing a way to conserve cardiovascular health? It's hard to see it that way when you are suffering from a headache.

One way to combat this is to use an antibacterial mouthwash, which decreases the concentration of the nitrate-reducing bacteria in your mouth. Vikas Kapil and his team from Queen Mary University in London showed in 2013 that this measure alone has the power to increase blood pressure, due to a 25 per cent decrease in nitrites (the precursor to nitric oxide) in the system. Or you could just stop eating bacon sandwiches.

Bar brawls

Let's end this trigger talk with a trip to the bar. We know that alcohol has various effects on our brain and the cerebrovascular system and that the resultant dehydration will cause a nasty headache. But is it a headache *trigger*? Alessandro Panconesi has trawled the literature for evidence of how this is reported. It turns out migraineurs don't report alcohol as a trigger any more than people who get tension headaches, and it's the same for men and women. Only 10 per cent of migraineurs report alcohol as a frequent trigger, but that might be because the rest of the migraine population avoid alcohol – a suggestion that seems to be backed up by consumption data.

Red wine is reported to be the villain of the piece although there is controversy because other studies implicate white wine and other drinks to a greater degree. Part of this is regional; people from the UK think that red wine is the worst; people from France and Italy think white wine and champagne are headache inducing (from my experience, I'm with them, but I do like a bit of bubbly). Perhaps this is more of a cultural narrative situation, then: because everybody in our social group says so, it must be true. Let's have a pint of science and discuss it.

There are a few suspects in the dock. Sulphites, tyramine, histamine and flavonoids in different forms of alcohol all stand accused. What the prosecutor needs to do is determine which of these have the power to induce headache (separate to the hangover or dehydration headache we talked about in Chapter 1) and if any of them are specific to migraine.

Rumour has it that sulphites are the biggest bad in wine. Sulphur dioxide is used in wine making as a preservative, since it's an efficient antimicrobial and an antioxidant. White wine contains a much higher concentration of sulphites than red wine, and dessert or sweet wines have higher concentrations again. There is a link between sulphites and histamine release, which in certain sensitive individuals could lead to breathlessness (more common in asthmatics), and this is caused by the sulphite's ability to release histamine, which narrows the bronchial tubes in your lungs, and is also on our trigger list for headache. Sulphites might also boost serotonin levels, so while our mood may improve while drinking, the serotonin is causing vasoconstriction. This may cause the neurovascular effects seen in migraine, but certainly causes rebound vasodilation, which will pull on the vessels' sensory nerve endings. Other than that, the evidence is scant; sulphites get off on a technicality: other foods (e.g. crisps, raisins, dried fruits, juices) contain 10 times the amount of sulphur dioxide than wine does but not that many people complain about those.

We've encountered tyramine in Chinese food and other places already, a repeat offender we might say, but the concentrations of tyramine in alcoholic beverages (and there is little variability between them) is very small and much less than that which is used by clinical scientists to prove tyramine has a vasoactive effect. So, tyramine in alcohol is released without charge. Tyramine in everything else, though, is still under suspicion.

Another repeat offender, histamine, doesn't get off so lightly, but mainly because it is a perpetrator of inflammatory responses with all alcoholic drinks and is egged on by the sulphites. It hangs in the red wine gang, having a greater concentration in your Malbec rather than your Muscadet. Even though we know it can provoke headache, and migraine in those who are prone, we still don't know if it is the driving factor of how alcohol triggers them.

Histamine's big brother in the red wine gang is the flavonoid. Flavonoids are naturally occurring in many plants and act as antioxidants; in alcohol they contribute to the colour, taste and mouthfeel of the drink. They are present in red wine in concentrations 23 times greater than those found in white wine, and include catechins (also found in tea and cocoa); anthocyanins, which give the wine its colour; and tannins, which contribute to the taste. The problem is, these particular flavonoids, which together represent 30 per cent of the flavonoid concentration in alcoholic beverages (of which there is more in red wine), are potent inhibitors of PST (phenolsulphotransferase)-P, which breaks down phenols, high concentrations of which can be toxic in the body, causing an immune inflammatory response.

Phenols in nature are powerful antiseptics and are the main ingredient in carbolic soap (my dad's favourite faux swear word). Nobody makes a habit of eating carbolic soap, but we do ingest phenols in the most common painkiller (among other drugs): paracetamol. Not being able to break phenols down means they hang around for longer and can have a harmful effect; inhibiting PST-P will lower the toxic threshold of the drug.

These effects of red wine and other alcoholic beverages are not, however, specific to migraine; they will trigger malaise in everyone. One point to note, though, is that in 1995 Mark Sandler from Queen Mary University in London found that there is a deficit of PST-P in the migraineurs he tested, meaning that alcohol may be a double whammy for them. In other words, not only do they have a deficit anyway, but alcohol will also lower it further. What's more, many alcoholic drinks have vasodilatory effects caused by the release of nitric oxide from the blood vessel walls and nerve endings through the action of the ethanol and histamine. And finally, ethanol itself promotes the release of CGRP, a prolific vasodilator and an agent that is already high in concentration in migraineurs.

Overall, though, the jury is out, still. For every study that says red wine is the baddy, others will say white. Wine has been linked to headache since the earliest medical encyclopaedias of Celcus at the beginning of the Common Era through to those of Paul of Aegina in the 7th century CE. There is therefore a historical precedence for this narrative. For every vasoconstriction mechanism, there is a vasodilatory one. And it's really difficult to show if it is what is in the beverage aside from the ethanol content that is acting as the trigger. It is also hard to be specific to migraine – all of these factors might cause any vascular headaches – but it is the special features of the migraneous brain that makes some people experience migraine from alcohol, though as Alessandro Panconesci found, only 10 per cent of migraineurs report alcohol as a specific trigger. The International Classification of Headache Disorders Criteria are strict; they say that migraine cannot be diagnosed when there are other possible causes for headache, including substance-induced toxicity. However, as we have seen, such toxicity may trigger migraine in the 'migraneous', but you won't be diagnosed as a migraineur based on your experience of an intoxication headache alone. Finally, we should also be mindful that these experiments involving different types of alcohol are very difficult to do. After the third glass of plonk, who really cares anymore?

Figure it out for yourself

Putting all of this together it is clear that there is a plethora of triggers for migraine. Some are major, such as patent foramen ovale, and some are relatively avoidable, such as nitrates. Some of them may sound familiar to you, some may be worth investigating; the individual differences here are vast and there is no one-size-fits-all solution. Prevention is better than cure of course, although there have been great strides in this field with the arrival of sumatriptan and Erenumab, both born of our clearer understanding of what is happening in the brain and body preceding and during a migraine episode and what made that happen; what is special about the migraneous brain. But you? You are inimitable. You have to identify your own triggers and you are uniquely placed to understand them. There are factors out there that wouldn't bother a regular person but make the migraineur much more susceptible to the induction of a headache. Working out which ones you can control and which ones you can't will allow you to wrestle the initiative back from this dreaded event.

8

What's Next?

I F YOU ARE ANYTHING like me, you might be a little
exasperated that we don't have a clear answer for how
to cure and indeed prevent all forms of headache by
now. After all, if we can trace back their origins deep into
our evolutionary history, in this day and age – 50 years
after we put men on the moon with no more technology
than is currently contained within your mobile phone –
why have we not solved this headache business? The
answer is complicated, by some things that we can see and
some things that we can't.

Let's first think about the things we can see. We know a lot
about headaches – how they present, what is happening in
the body during their course, how people experience them.
Medical, clinical and molecular science enquiry has grown
up around the issue so that we have a better understanding
now than ever before about the molecules like CGRP that
might have an influence, right up to physical processes
like cortical spreading depolarisation. Sure, there've been
false starts and avenues that turned into dead ends (MSG,
anyone?) but treatments to interact with these levels have
been born and have been successfully deployed in the past.
But science, like lots of other things, such as running a
business for example, suffers from the aperture problem,
with people only focused on a tiny pixel of the overall

picture. That can give you a really false impression of what the whole picture looks like. For example, if you were to look a square centimetre of your face in a photo, would you be able to identify yourself? You might not even think that square came from a face – it could just as well come from a paper bag (entirely preferable in my case). But if you zoom out, it begins to become apparent that you are looking at a face and that that face is yours.

In the investigation of headache it is really important that we do this kind of zooming out; sense checking our purpose in a way. We must get our molecular scientists, together with our physiologists, flow dynamists (who look at what makes blood flow in a turbulent or smooth way), computer scientists, statisticians, clinicians, neuro-scientists, psychologists, physiotherapists and indeed patients involved in our next stage of enquiry. This interdisciplinary approach is the future. It will ensure that we ask the right questions and interpret the answers in the realm of human experience and reality. We can also borrow from other disciplines. One of the great tickle points of my life has been following a story that has seeped into a load of other fields, including migraine.

The rhythm of life is a powerful beat

It all started with a Columbian neuroscientist called Rodolfo Llinás and his team at New York University in the late 1990s. Having spent years working on how single neurons talk to each other in various parts of the brain and looking at how neurotransmitters are released in the giant squid synapse, he then changed his focus. He is a brilliant example of how to change the scale that you are working on.

Magnetoencephalography (MEG)

This is a technique that marries the best qualities of functional imaging, allowing you to know *where* something is happening, with the brilliant specificity in time that physiological recording like electroencephalography (EEG) gives us so that we also know *when* something is happening.

What the MEG machine does is detect and decode the magnetic fields that our brains are generating. Wherever there is an electrical current, and our brains are full of those, there will be a magnetic field associated with it. It is the principal of electromagnetism as discovered by Michael Faraday, an English scientist way back in 1831. Google him. He looks like your quintessential mad scientist (based on historical pictures of scientists, I often thought I wasn't going to make it unless I was somewhat bald, with copious facial hair and wore a frock coat) but he utterly changed the game around energy, our understanding of it and how we can harness it. Not only are we surrounded by exemplars of his theories in our daily lives (every time we switch an electrical appliance on, for example) but his work was also the basis of transcranial magnetic stimulation (TMS) and MEG.

Rodolfo zoomed out his lens from looking at these almost microscopic properties to investigate how neurons communicate across the brain. Using MEG, he realised that in Parkinson's patients, he was seeing a pattern of activity coming from the motor cortex (the bit that makes us move) in exact synchronicity with the twitch that his patients exhibited: about three twitches a second. But he also saw this pattern in another place in the brain, namely the thalamus, which sits underneath the cortex. There are connections from the thalamus to every bit of the cortex and back again and so these 'thalamocortical loops' are involved in everything that we do. As Rodolfo was interested in a movement disorder (Parkinson's disease) he tracked the motor thalamocortical loop and noticed that the thalamus set the pace for what happens in the cortex. It turns out that abnormal rhythms can happen in any of the thalamocortical loops, affecting any function, and that this symptom is apparent in a wide variety of brain-based disorders. The thalamus generates the signal to the cortex based on the input it is getting from elsewhere, so it is not necessarily the cause of the problem, but its reaction to it potentiates the symptoms.

This knowledge gives us an incredible opportunity. If the screwy signals coming from the thalamus cause the symptoms through their action on the cortex then can we play with those? In the early days, Daniel Jeanmonod, a neurosurgeon from Zurich, destroyed little areas of the thalamus thought to be involved in the motor loop in Parkinson's patients on the proviso that no signals are better than screwy signals. However, the side effects were massive; it was just too hard to be that precise 20 years ago and it's not like these neurons looked any different to any others. A major advance was made when Daniel started to put electrodes into the area to 'listen' for the abnormal signals, and then he could destroy the area that was sending those out. Outcomes were better, twitching decreased or ceased, but it was still fraught with risk.

But what if instead of destroying an area, we could actually set the pace of the neural firing from this very slow rate to a more normal faster rate? We can do it with the heart when the natural pacemaker of the electrical activity that causes heart contractions fails, and now we can with the brain, too. It's called deep brain stimulation and can have value in a variety of disorders, including motor disorders like Parkinson's and dystonia (where all of the muscles are tensed up), obsessive compulsive disorder, Tourette's syndrome, tinnitus, migraine and cluster headache. The effects are instant and striking. The battery for the pacemaker is fitted under the skin in the chest and if you switch off the stimulator by passing a magnetic field over it, the symptoms instantly return. You can even have a stimulator in both sides of the brain controlling your symptoms on both sides of the body. It really is life-changing.

Having these slow signals coming from the thalamus means that the area of cortex, the eye of the storm, that it feeds is getting very abnormal inputs, making it act irrationally. Even worse, instead of the cortex receiving constant steady input, it is now receiving bursts of activity in an on/off fashion. The usual way the cortex tamps down on activity breaks down, meaning that the area becomes overactivated, setting up a wave of excitation radiating out from the eye of the storm. As we saw in Chapter 6, this description sounds very like the wave of excitation we see at the beginning of the migraine attack, followed closely by the wave of depressed activity. In the case of migraine, we still don't know for sure where the cause of the thalamocortical effect lies – there could be a number of reasons, as we have discussed. It could be that the overactive visual cortex of the migraineur feeds back to the thalamus, which tries to correct this with slower signals back to the cortex. Regardless, Thalamocortical

Dysrhythmia, as Rodolfo Llinás called it, is certainly complicit in the migraine experience.

This means that for those whom medicine doesn't help, there is another way. Deep brain stimulation to reset the communication pathway between the thalamus and the cortex is a credible last resort and shows some good efficacy. There is positive progress here for cluster headache, too. It seems more certain that it is regions of the hypothalamus that are to blame here, and these regions then project to the thalamus. Harith Akram, a neurosurgeon from University College London, has identified a good area of stimulation is an area in which the trigeminal and other areas involved in pain perception meet with the hypothalamus, towards the back side of the hypothalamus. In 2017, he reported a 30 per cent reduction in pain, so with even greater precision afforded by advances in neurosurgical techniques and our understanding of the underlying neuroscience, this option can only become more credible.

The magnet and the mind

There are ways that we can play with the activity of the outermost layer of the brain that is responsible for actioning the symptoms we can see and this has had some importance, particularly for people who experience migraine. I've mentioned already that transcranial magnetic stimulation (TMS) can be used to briefly and reversibly switch on an area of neurons inside the brain. This involves holding a magnetic coil that discharges a magnetic pulse to the skull. It just feels like a tap on your head but it passes really easily through the skull into the brain tissue below. Through Michael Faraday's electromagnetic induction, this magnetic pulse induces an electrical current in the brain and this causes action potentials to happen. In the lab, I can use this to work out not just what an area of your brain is doing but also when it is talking to other regions. Various treatments have resulted that the patient can use at home either as a preventive measure against migraine attack or as soon as the migraine experience starts.

The most popular form of treatment being recommended at the moment is to deliver two pulses 30 seconds apart using a device the patient holds to the back of their head. I've worked with TMS for 25 years, so you're going to have to forgive me for being a little sceptical. The kinds of protocols we use in the lab are much more precise, both with respect to where we deliver pulses in the brain and how powerful they are. They have to be, in order to find out anything at all, because the brain really sees what I am doing with my TMS coil as a bit of nuisance noise. Holding a device imprecisely to the back of the head and tickling the brain with a couple of pulses, each with mere milliseconds of effect in the brain and expecting it to kick-start the area into a more synchronous activity seems like a bit of a leap to me. Having said all of that, there has been a randomised controlled trial. Of the included 164 people who experience migraine with aura, 39 per cent of patients were pain-free two hours after treatment in comparison with 22 per cent after placebo treatment. Results also showed that 29 per cent had no recurrence or need for any further treatment after 24 hours in comparison with 16 per cent of people who had the placebo treatment. There may be something there. The use of TMS doesn't preclude any other treatments though and so it could be used as another combat tool in the box.

Scale has also been important in the development of a different non-drug intervention, this time focusing on manipulating the activity of a nerve that is quite accessible on either side of the neck. The vagus nerve is the tenth cranial nerve, and you have one on each side of your body. Need your heart to beat faster? No problem. Need your blood vessels to dilate or contract? That's your vagus nerve too. It also tells your brain what it has done through sensory feedback and carries pain signals from the nociceptors or pain receptors up to the brain. Knowing this, transcutaneous vagal nerve stimulation (tVNS) has been developed to interact with this rather peripheral node in the pain network. Electrical currents are released from a device the size of a mobile phone that is held to the neck for about 90 seconds, and the stimulation of the vagus nerve seems to modulate the firing rate of the pain neurons in the trigeminal pathway. This then has a knock-on effect for how our brains perceive pain, by increasing the inhibition that damps down the pain response. This treatment seems to have good efficacy, particularly in people who suffer from cluster headaches and who can't tolerate injected sumatriptan and in whom oral sumatriptan has no effect.

What's good for the goose may not be good for the gander

Another thing that we can see is the variability between all of us; we have to start including this knowledge in how we decide how efficacious our treatments are at an individual level. When drugs are put through clinical trials, the smallest amount of variability is preferable so that we can get the cleanest possible answer as to whether the drug works or not, and whether or not it is safe. But we only get to this stage after a number of other steps. Funding has to be secured to develop the drug, either from the national research councils or from the pharma industry. Once a drug has reached the point at which it can be administered, it is then required, by law, to be tested in two animal models, usually rodents and dogs, before it can get to human clinical trials. Now, I have known many humans who have acted like rats and dogs, but as a comparative physiologist, I know that they are entirely different. If the drug fails in curing these animals of whatever illness has been inflicted upon them to test the drug, then the science goes back to the drawing board. But what if the drug would have worked in humans, and doesn't work in animals because their physiology is different? And, on top of that, there are many examples of drugs working in animals that have no effect or even dire consequences in humans.

Shouldn't we find a better way of testing drugs meant for humans by replacing the need for animals at this stage? Not only would we do better science, perhaps arriving at answers much more quickly than the animal detour allowed us to, but we would get to not inflict all manner of illness on our fellow custodians of the planet. I am happy to report that great strides are being made on the science side of this issue. In my post-doctoral years I was funded by a wonderful charity called Animal Free Research UK, which support scientists young and old to find alternatives to animal testing. Before the advent of TMS, the kinds of questions we were answering would have been addressed using lesions to monkey brains. That certainly wasn't my bag, so I was honoured to be part of the constructive solution, finding a credible and valid alternative to this practice.

The next step is to change the law that requires animal testing before clinical trials and prove that we can have as much confidence in the human-based replacement as we would in the animal model. Who knows what useful treatments we have missed out on because they didn't work on animals? Scientific discovery is hard enough without creating blind alleys for ourselves along the way.

The clinical trials themselves are another issue. There has been much concern recently that many are done with men, because the cyclical nature of the release of female hormones muddies the waters somewhat. To determine if this is a real phenomenon, Geert Labots from Leiden in the Netherlands looked at 38 drugs (and the 185,000+ people who participated in their trials) that had been approved by the FDA in the USA to see if there was any difference there. Sure enough, in Phase 1 trials, where scientists are trying to investigate side effects and what happens to the drug in the body, there was a difference, with only 22 per cent of participants being female. These studies tend to be small, involving only 20–50 people, but nevertheless the possibility of progressing to Phase 2 is contingent upon these results. Phase 2 includes more than 100 people and finds out more about side effects and how well the treatment works. Phase 3 could include thousands of people and is randomised; this is where the new drug is compared with the standard treatment to see if it infers any advantage at all. Phases 2 and 3 had a much better gender divide, approaching parity between the sexes. The lynchpin is Phase 1 though, so this factor is certainly something to think about in the future.

And it is not just what sex you are that makes a difference. If you are a night owl or an early bird, you should modulate when you take your drugs. For example, if you have high blood pressure, taking your medication at night will have a maximal and lasting effect on the system that controls blood pressure, the renin–angiotension–aldosterone system that activates during night-time sleep. This is called chronotherapy (from the Greek *khronos*-meaning 'time'); the right dose of the right drug at the right time leads to a more effective outcome and often then requires smaller doses.

The dosage of drugs is currently the same for every adult no matter what size you are or how fast your metabolism is. And don't even get me started on co-morbidities. If you suffer from headache but you also have an arrhythmia and a pain in your big toe, we don't tend to put these things together as being causative of each other (such as gout caused by circulatory problems). Most of this time, our various aches and pains are pretty random, especially as we get older, but sometimes, pulling the lens out of the condition that the patient presents with will help diagnose a headache as not just a headache for headache's sake, but a circulatory problem that could be best tackled some other manner. In the same way as thinking about the individual's circadian rhythm for optimal treatment, putting together information from different fields leads to a treatment that is more personalised and effective.

So what about the things that we can't really see? How do we put all our lives together into some kind of narrative that will illuminate the factor or factors that are causing you to get headaches? If there was ever a time to poke around in the wardrobe of your life, this would be it. Take every piece out, see if the moths have got to it. If they have, recycle it; take what you have learned and let it go. Even if the moths haven't enjoyed the fabric, are you really going to wear it again? As you will probably know, the best way to do this is to keep a diary. This doesn't have to be a Dear Diary diary, but merely a record of your day. What you ate, how much exercise you got in and when you did it, what you drank, how you felt at different points in the day, what emotional pressures you had on you – that kind of thing. People tend to only do this when they feel awful, but it is so important to have the contrast with when you felt well. You need to look at all of the factors that affect your health, both physical and mental. And just like Kate Blackmore, the paediatric ENT surgeon we met in Chapter 3, we can become detectives but in this case of our own lives. We all have triggers, some of which we can watch out for and manage, such as dehydration, posture or flashy lights. There are some, though, as we have seen, that we won't know about and the first thing we notice are the symptoms of headache. Knowing that your headache doesn't just live in your head, that its effect and often its cause happens in your body, or your behaviour, should help you be more holistic in your approach.

Pain means something, take it seriously.

Endnotes

CHAPTER 2

1 Usually my class was in January, the same month as Maya did most of her data collection. There is a theory that you can only experience ice cream headache if it is warm. Well, Ontario, Canada, isn't the warmest place on the planet in January (Maya said it rarely gets above 0 degrees centigrade, which is freezing to me, who grew up in a temperate climate warmed by the Gulf Stream) but Maya didn't do her experiments outside so presumably room temperature negates this argument as a point of contrast. So both Maya and I would have run our experiments in relatively warm environments, making ice cream headache more likely.

2 Dublin-born, like myself, Robert Smith studied at the medical school of my alma mater, Trinity College Dublin, during World War II, graduating in 1946. He subsequently moved to Surrey in the UK to practise there, and following a stint tending to the medical needs of the British Army and their families in post-war Germany, he became one of the first trainees in general practice when the National Health Service (NHS) was created. He went on to set up schools of family medicine in Guy's Hospital in London, Chapel Hill in North Carolina and finally, the University of Cincinnati, where he also set up the Cincinnati Headache Center. In the middle of all of this, he was researching various aspects of pain. Hence the ice chips.

CHAPTER 3

1 White-water kayaking is a winter sport. In a kayak, I would wear a rash vest, swim shorts, a wetsuit, a cagoule with watertight seals at the neck and wrists, a buoyancy aid and

dry pants with watertight seals at the ankle and waist, wetsuit boots, a skull cap and a helmet, in addition to a spray deck that attached to the cockpit in the kayak to keep my legs relatively dry. If I had my way, that's what I would have worn to the waterpark (which was indoors, incidentally) but I have only so much resilience to people staring.

2　I had cause to be very glad that chlorine had been used in the pool when the little boy beside me in the wave pool later that day shouted to his mum: 'I need a wee... Never mind...' as a look of sheer relief overtook his features. I couldn't move away fast enough. I actually couldn't as I had torn my watershorts and underlying swimsuit when I had got stuck on that slide and was concerned for my modesty.

3　Pneumococcus was discovered independently in 1881 by both well-known chemist Louis Pasteur in France and a US Army physician, George Sternberg. It is a Gram-positive bacteria and looks like little blades made up of elongated spheres or 'cocci' (singular: coccus) and will often pair up to become 'diplococci', by which name it was known until 1920. They are particularly beautiful in three dimensions, where they look like chains of spheres.

4　A number of cases have been documented whereby certain people develop a triad whereby they get asthma, sinus and polyps with aspirin sensitivity. Thirty per cent of people with asthma and polyps have a sensitivity to aspirin (but also ibuprofen). This combined response probably has something to do with the aspirin's activity blocking the prostaglandin immune response but the exact causes are not yet known.

CHAPTER 4

1　Social psychologists like Mario Weick call this 'the planning fallacy'. People in positions of power, or those who need things done by other people, tend to underestimate how long it will take to get things done. It's not because they are inept, it's because they view their task at hand as unique and think that whatever may have happened in similar circumstances previously, things will be better this time around. It's also related to the fact that they just don't think about all the other things that people have on their plates to do as well as what they have asked for. They are more focused on the intended outcome and not all of the steps and cogs in the wheel to get to that outcome. So, timescales slip. Unless they are surrounded by superhumans, which simply feeds the fallacy.

2   You might also take beta-blockers if your heart is beating too fast because of a different underlying condition such as an overactive thyroid gland. Your thyroid hormone is important in how fast your metabolism goes and is usually tightly controlled through communication between the hypothalamus, pituitary and thyroid gland. The most common thyroid condition is autoimmune, where your own immune system attacks the gland, which rather counter intuitively makes it bigger, producing more thyroid hormone. Patients with this condition have really high resting heart rates, sometimes well in excess of 100 beats per minute. They breathe quickly and talk fast and have the energy of an entire under-10s football team. Cognitively, they feel rushed and stressed and find it hard to grasp a thought before it flies out of their head. Part of this is because of the interpretation of that beating heart and fast breathing as threat by the brain. Beta-blockers calm this down as they do for the emotional causes of stress in the body by dealing with the bodily effect, but not the emotional causes.

Chapter 5

1   It wasn't actually recognised as its own class of headache until 1998, having been lumped in with migraine up until then. However, it was first extensively described centuries before in 1694 by a Dutch physician called Nicolaas Tulp.

2   It's probably clear by now that I am no fan of non-descriptive terms, preferring 'apoplexy', 'subarachnoid haemorrhage' or 'ischemia' to 'stroke', for example. The reason we call it stroke today is due to the influence of religion. Because it

changes your life quickly and often irrevocably, it was seen as 'the stroke of the hand of God'. Stroke, as a term, stuck.

3   Perhaps my preference for the term cluster is determined by this rather groovy nominative.

4   Interestingly, there are HCRTR2 receptors all over the brain that ensure these complex behaviours are carried out, and so orexin has a reputation for integrating multiple physiological functions.

5   It is too early to tell what effect vaping will have on nicotine dosing as this is a habit that is not as easy to keep track of, because it is not packaged in the same way as cigarettes.

6   Schools that have reset their timetables accordingly have reported dramatic decreases in truancy and improvements in student well-being and mental health. There is no point in telling a teenager to go to bed; their body just isn't ready. They live in a different time zone.

7   Of course, we didn't know this in Horton's time; back then it was thought that they were caused by stress and bad diet. It took until 1982 for Barry Marshall and Robin Warren, two Australian physicians, to prove that stomach ulcers were caused by bacteria, and the scientific and medical establishment only started listening in 1984. But listen they did when finally, in an act of complete and utter frustration, Robin drank a solution swimming with the bacteria Barry and he had painstakingly isolated. Lo and behold, he developed a stomach ulcer! He then treated himself with antibiotics and made a full recovery. Part of the medical community didn't believe it ('if it is caused by bacteria then why haven't we seen this before?' being a common complaint) and part of it was utterly agog. For this reason, it was the early 1990s before the pharmaceutical industry and clinical practice started to treat ulcers systemically in this way, with the first targeted antibiotic coming on the market in 1995. In 2005, Barry Marshall and Robin Warren accepted their Nobel Prize in Physiology or Medicine for work that had started with the observation under the microscope of a high load of bacteria

in the gut of an ulcer sufferer and their ability to draw the correct conclusion.

8   A biologist herself, Lisa Kudrow published a paper with her dad in 1994 debunking the idea, at least in California, that more left-handed people suffered from cluster headaches than right-handers.

9   In his spare time, Lance also likes to spot the neurobiology lessons in the works of Shakespeare, such as the description of Othello's epilepsy by the treacherous Iago in Act 4 Scene 1!

CHAPTER 6

1   The myelin sheath is what is attacked and destroyed in multiple sclerosis (MS), thus demonstrating its enormous value to us. In people who suffer from MS, movement and eventually thought and breathing become impossible over time.

2   A term preferred by radiologists to describe this low blood volume; *oligaemia* is borrowed from the Greek for 'uncountable'.

3   Ti'u was the specific evil spirit of the headache, represented in the Mesopotamian pictorial language or logography by *sag-gig*, or head illness. It depicted Ti'u pointing to a person's head, suggesting horrendous headaches with after-effects of dry lips, loss of appetite and urination.

4   The thalamus is my second-favourite area of the brain after the hypothalamus (which sits below the thalamus, as the name suggests). *Thalamus* is Latin for 'inner chamber' or 'bedroom', which is apt given that the thalamus in our brain sets the activity, or firing, rate of the rest of the brain. It literally slows everything down when we want to go to sleep and starts it all up again to wake up.

5   These migraineurs can't suppress their grins when they tell me about this – they know they are the lucky ones. For example, 62-year-old Mary told me: 'I don't generally talk about it in my group of friends. They all get headaches, we're accountants! But people get so jealous. I see it as my

reward for coming out the other side!' Since dopamine is the neurotransmitter that mediates the reward centres of the brain, her choice of words couldn't have been more prescient.

CHAPTER 7

1   Hippocrates was born on the island of Kos, Greece, in 460 BCE and reached the ripe old age of 85, living through the Classical Greek period. A philosopher and a physician, he and his followers turned away from the idea that illness was caused by spirits or gods and other superstitions, believing instead that patients must be individually and closely observed in order to come up with a rational treatment plan. The whole patient should be considered, and their diet, sleep, exercise and work should be monitored as these were deemed important factors in causing and therefore reversing imbalances in the humours. This approach is very much reflected in our modern interdisciplinary enquiry, although through the ages humanity subsequently fell into a one-size-fits-all category.

2   At least for people who like to think about the evolution of our thoughts about how anything happens in our body, how we experience it and how it guides our behaviour.

3   As Hippocrates is accepted as the father of medicine, Thomas is the father of neurology, being the first to coin the term in the first textbook of clinical neurology, which he wrote. He discovered the nature of our reflexes and also described the Circle of Willis, a central and indeed vital cross-connection of arteries that serves the brain and all of its structures. Thomas imagined that the vague, occult-like communication that served the Greek 'sympathy' was actually based in a neurophysiological framework, leading him to predict many of the findings that proved his theories at late as the 19th century.

4   Psychological study of the migrainous syndrome, Herman Selinsky, *Bulletin of the New York Academy of Medicine*, 1939, Vol. 15, pp.757–763.

5   This role was to be the reason why Gregor's experiments had to stop; the administrative burden of running the monastery

was too great to allow anything else. It was ever thus in the academic career. He had chosen to become a friar at least in part because it meant his education was paid for and his living expenses were taken care of, letting him carry out his scientific enquiries, but his fast-track promotion made sure his plan backfired somewhat.

6   Do I need to explain why? I once reached out to the legend that is Dolly Parton over Twitter to ask her if she knew this. She didn't respond of course, but somebody told me she did in fact know, and that she wanted to get a jumper made from Dolly's wool. Dollywool! I don't know if she ever got it.

7   The word Jaagsiekte is Afrikaans for 'chase' (*jaag*) and 'sickness' (*siekte*) because affected sheep are constantly out of breath, as if they had been chased.

8   A Chinese team, lead by Yiqing Huang, gave it a bash in 2017, but it is not usually the norm; one gene tends to be followed in one family.

9   Three weeks later I walked into the house and immediately clapped eyes on that stripy top again. A wave of nausea instantly ensued (pretty sure it was in reaction to the shirt). So, if spousal sartorial choices are not grounds for divorce (they are not, I checked), perhaps throwing up on your spouse is.

10 Sometimes two are released, leading to fraternal twins if both are fertilised by a visiting sperm cell over the next 24 hours, and even multiples beyond two (those are called 'the motherload').

Glossary

Action potential: the way in which a neuron becomes active, creating an electrical signal that then passes down the neuron.

Adrenaline: also known as epinephrine, adrenaline is a hormone released by the adrenal glands and is very important in the fight-or-flight response of the sympathetic nervous system.

Amygdala: an almond shaped brain structure, one on each side. It is very important in how we produce and perceive emotions.

Aneurysm: a bulb in a blood vessel which causes turbulent flow of the blood. They happen most commonly in the brain and in the abdomen.

Antibodies: immune markers that we raise having been exposed to a bacteria or virus. It means we can combat them quickly next time and so are immune to their charms.

Autonomic: involuntary and unconscious

Autonomic nervous system: All of the bodily functions over which we have no conscious awareness are controlled by the autonomic nervous system. The cardiovascular system, the endocrine system, the digestive system and lots of others come under its control.

Axon: the part of the neuron that protrudes from the cell body and takes the signal to the next neuron or a muscle.

Axon hillock: the area of the axon that decides whether there has been enough net excitation (over inhibition) caused in its neuron by all of the other neurons synapsing onto it.

Bioabsorbable: a substance that the body can absorb to become part of its tissue.

Bronchospasm: narrowing of the airways in the lungs.

Cerebrovascular system: the blood vessels that bring blood to and away from the brain.

Cilia: tiny little hairs that are present on the surface of some cells in the body.

218

Ciliated pseudostratified columnar epithelial cells: cells that are found
   lining the sinuses. They look like layers under the microscope
   but there is actually only one layer, they are just different sizes.
   They have cilia on their outer surface to move the mucus along.
Cocci: any bacteria that has a sphere-like shape will have a name
   ending in *–coccus (singular)* or *cocci (plural).*
Coccobacilli: any bacteria that has a shape in between the
   spherical cocci and the rod-like bacilli.
Concentration gradient: as you pour cordial into a glass of water, it will
   be more concentrated at the bottom initially. Over time it will
   spread to be equally distributed in the glass. The concentration
   gradient is driving this movement from areas of high
   concentration to areas of low. It is the same principle by which
   people distribute themselves in lecture theatres, and bathrooms.
Cortical spreading depolarisation: a wave of excitation, or
   depolarisation, passes over the cortex of the brain in migraine.
Cortical spreading depression: The wave of excitation (cortical spreading
   depolarisation) seen in migraine is followed by cortical spreading
   depression, or a wave of relative inactivity (depression).
Cortisol: a hormone released from the adrenal gland which
   regulates our metabolism and immune response and is heavily
   involved in our response to stress (physical and mental).
Depolarisation: the insides of our neurons are more negative
   with respect to the outside. The inside and outside are polar
   opposites, or polarised. Depolarisation is when the inside of the
   cells gets more positive (so that the two sides are less polarised).
Diuretics: any chemical agent that makes us urinate more. Coffee
   and alcohol are the most common.
Dyspnoea: shortness of breath
Endocrine system: the system that regulates the body's activity
   via hormones.
Endogenous opioids: our own natural painkillers, they act in the
   pain centres of the brain to dampen our perception of pain.
Endorphins: these endogenous opioids are released to relieve stress
   and pain in the body.
Endoscopic: the use of a tiny camera on the end of a very thin
   tube so that structures can be seen inside our body.

Enzyme: any substance that speeds up a chemical reaction.

Epigenetics: the study of how our environment can change how our genes are switched on and off (and therefore what proteins are produced, or not as the case may be).

Episodic cluster pain: if you have a break of from one month up to several years between a cluster headache attack, this will be diagnosed as episodic.

Epithelial cells: surface cells that separate the outside from the inside. They are found in skin, blood vessels, the urinary tract, the respiratory system, the urinary system and organs.

Gamma amino butyric acid (GABA): the brain's main inhibitory neurotransmitter.

Ganglion: a grouping of neurons, and their cell bodies.

Genome-wide association studies (GWAS): an observational study in which the whole genome is investigated or variants between individuals to see if any of these variants can be associated with a trait or disorder.

Glial cells: support cells in the nervous system. They wrap around neurons to make signals go faster (the myelin sheath) and they mop up toxins and other substances that may harm the neuron or its action.

Glutamate: the most common excitatory neurotransmitter in the brain.

Goblet cells: a kind of epithelium cell that releases mucus.

Histamine: the first responders to tissue injury, histamine drives inflammation and also acts in the brain to keep us alert.

Hypothalamus: the endocrine system's puppet master, the hypothalamus is a structure under the cerebral cortex that reacts to the concentration of circulating hormones to either make sure more are produced and released or that production is stopped.

Hypovolemia: too little volume, usually associated with blood volume.

Immunoglobulins: antibodies produced by white blood cells that recognise and stick to antigens such as bacteria or viruses, but also allergens so that they can be destroyed effectively.

Inhibitory neurons: neurons that release inhibitory neurotransmitter meaning that activity of the neurons they connect with will be suppressed.

Ion: a charged particle, either positive or negative.

Ischemia: a lack of blood flow due to a restriction of blood supply (usually a blockage of some sort).

Limbic system: the emotional system of the brain, the limbic system comprises a number of loosely connected areas that allow us to recognise and produce appropriate emotions in the setting in which we find ourselves.

Lysozymes: organelles inside each cell body that contain enzymes that will kill the cell if the lysosome bursts (if the cell isn't functioning correctly, for example.)

Magnetoencephalography: a neuroscientific technique that allows us to map what is happening in the brain in addition to where and when. It works by detecting the magnetic fields that the electrical activity in the brain result in.

Mast cells: these cells live just under the epithelium and release their contents, including histamine and other factors that trigger the immune system when the tissue comes under attack.

Meninges: the covering of the brain between the grey matter of the cerebral cortex and the skull.

Myelin sheath: the coating that glial cells provide by wrapping themselves around the axon to allow it to pass the electrical signal (action potential) down its length quicker.

Neurochemicals: any chemicals that interact with neurons. These may be neurotransmitters but also chemicals that control how well neurotransmitters work.

Neurons: nerve cells. There are many forms but the main two are motor (taking information from the brain to the body) and sensory (taking information from the body to the brain). The brain is also full of interneurons allowing different areas of the brain to talk to each other.

Neuropeptide: small protein-like molecules that influence how neurons and other cells in the body work.

Neutrophils: white blood cells that are important in our response to damage, infection or other stressors.

Nociceptors: pain receptors that are sensory neurons that detect potentially damaging stimuli. It is only perceived as pain though once this signal has been processed in the brain.

Nucleus: the brain of the cell, this is the organelle in the cell body where all of our chromosomes live.

Oxytocin: made in the hypothalamus, this is the bonding hormone. It is released after childbirth and at the dawn of new relationships.

Pain gating: a way of lessening the impact of pain signals by reducing our ability to perceive them. Examples include rubbing it better (the brain will listen to the mechanical signal over the pain signal) or distraction.

Pain receptors: or nociceptors; sensory neurons that detect potentially damaging stimuli.

Parasympathetic system: the rest and digest part of the autonomic nervous system that calms the body down after a period of stress. Also active when the body is maintaining calm.

Patent foramen ovale: a hole in the septum (the barrier between the right and left of the heart) of the atrium which has not closed up properly after birth.

Periodic cluster pain: when cluster headaches occur at the same time of year.

Phosphenes: spots of light that can be detected by stimulating either the brain or the retina directly (by pressing your finger to your closed eyelid).

Photic sneeze: sneezing caused by exposure to bright light caused by cross wiring in your brain.

Piloerection: when the hairs on your arm stand on end.

Pituitary gland: the puppet of the hypothalamus, this master gland sits just below the hypothalamus and sends signals to the other glands of the body to produce or release their hormones. It also directly releases oxytocin and anti-diuretic hormone, which acts on the kidneys. Both are made in the hypothalamus.

Population genetics: the study of genetic variation within a population allowing us to see how this changes over time.

Post-nasal drip: when mucus runs down the back of your nose into your throat.

Postsynaptic membrane: The membrane of a dendrite or cell body that comes after the synapse. This is where the neurotransmitter that has been dumped into the gap (synapse) by the previous neurons binds with proteins to open ion channels starting off the electrical activity again.

Preoptic nucleus: an area of the hypothalamus very important in temperature regulation and sexual activity.

Primary motor cortex: the area of the brain just in front of the central sulcus in the frontal cortex that controls all of the fine movements our body has to do.

Primary viral infection: a virus that was able to attack and compromise our body in its fit state.

Primary visual cortex: the first area of the visual system where light is processed into lines. It is located at the very back of the brain in the occipital cortex.

Proprioception: the sense by which we know what the muscles and joints of our body are doing.

Prostaglandins: little lipid molecules that are important in the inflammatory response to tissue damage.

Referred pain: pain that you feel as coming from one place when actually it originates in another. It is caused by the pain signals from the two places being lumped together and our brain is not able to discriminate between the two (e.g. pain signals from the heart are perceived as pain in the left arm).

Rhinitis: inflammation inside the nose.

Rhinovirus: infections that cause the common cold.

Scotoma: a small, usually circular, blind spot in the visual field (the space we can see).

Serotonin: a neurotransmitter important in emotional regulation; also known as the happy hormone.

Serotonin agonist: an agonist is any molecule that acts just like or causes the same effect as a neurotransmitter, in this case serotonin.

Sinus: the sinuses are small, hollow spaces behind the cheekbones and forehead that connect to the nose. The term sinus is also interchangeable with sinusitis.

Sinusitis: inflammation of the lining of the sinuses.

Somatosensation: our ability to feel mechanical and temperature stimuli on the surface of the body.

Somatosensory cortex: an area of the brain just behind the central sulcus in the parietal lobe where all the sensory information coming from the body is processed so that we know what we are feeling and where.

Sub-mucosa: the layer of tissue beneath the mucous membrane. Here, we find blood vessels and nerves among other things.

Suprachiasmatic nucleus: an area of the hypothalamus that responds to light input to create our daily circadian rhythm.

Sympathetic system: the fight or flight part of the autonomic nervous system, it marshals our resources to allow us to deal effectively with threat or stress.

Synaptic clefts: the gap between neurons that are communicating with each other. It is where the neurotransmitters are released into and so houses the chemical part of electrochemical conduction.

Terminal bouton: the last part of the neuron. Arrival of an action potential here causes an influx of calcium into the bouton, which triggers the vesicles to fuse with the terminal membrane to dump their contents out into the synaptic cleft.

Thalamocortical loops: reciprocal loops of connected neurons and areas that function together to bring about a behaviour such as movement, vision, thinking, etc. The thalamus acts as the pacemaker.

Thalamus: the grand relay centre of the brain, all sensory and motor signals pass through here on their way to the cortex and often back again as part of thalamocortical loops.

Trigeminal nerve: responsible for sensation in the face and also movements such as biting and chewing.

Trigeminal pathway: this pathway carries pain, touch and temperature information to the brain from the face.

Vascular system: any system that involves blood vessels – for example cardiovascular system in the heart or cerebrovascular system in the brain.

Vasoactive: any chemical or agent that can interact and change the diameter or action of blood vessels.

Vasoconstrictor: any chemical or agent that can narrow the diameter of blood vessels.

Vasodilation: any chemical or agent that can widen the diameter of blood vessels.

Vesicles: tiny pouches that contain a substance (such as neurotransmitter vesicles).

Zona incerta: an area beneath the cortex of the brain that is involved in the perception of the affective component of pain (i.e. how bad the pain is) as opposed to the sensory component of pain (what it feels like). Activity here is coincident with chronic pain in the absence of a sensory stimulus.

Further Reading

Ellison, A. (2012) *Getting Your Head Around the Brain* (London: Palgrave).

Hari, J. (2019) *Lost Connections: Why You're Depressed and How to Find Hope* (London: Bloomsbury).

Rapport, R. (2005) *Nerve Endings: The Discovery of the Synapse* (New York: W. W. Norton and Company).

Rutherford, A. (2017) *A Brief History of Everyone Who Ever Lived: The Stories in Our Genes* (London: Weidenfeld & Nicolson).

Wilmut, I., Campbell, K. and Tudge, C. (2000) *The Second Creation: Dolly and the Age of Biological Control* (London: Headline).

Selected References

CHAPTER 1

Bushra, R., & Aslam, N. (2010) 'An overview of clinical pharmacology of Ibuprofen,' *Oman Medical Journal*, 25(3): 155–1661. https://DOI.org/10.5001/omj.2010.49.

CHAPTER 2

Kaczorowski M., Kaczorowski, J. (2002) 'Ice cream evoked headaches (ICE-H) study: Randomised trial of accelerated versus cautious ice cream eating regimen,' *BMJ*, 325: 1445.

Blatt, M. M., Falvo, M., Jasien, J., Deegan, B., Ó Laighin, G., and Serrador, J. (2012) 'Cerebral vascular blood flow changes during 'Brain Freeze,'' *The FASEB Journal*, 26(1_supplement): 685.4–685.4.

CHAPTER 3

Medina, E., Romero, C., Brenes M., and De Castro, A. (2007) 'Antimicrobial activity of olive oil, vinegar, and various beverages against foodborne pathogens,' *Journal of Food Protection*, 70(5): 1194–1199.

Arshad S. H., Karmaus, W., Raza, A., Kurukulaaratchy, R. J., Matthews, S. M., Holloway, J. W., Sadeghnejad, A., Zhang, H., Roberts, G., Ewart S. L. (2012) 'The effect of parental allergy on childhood allergic diseases depends on the sex of the child,' *Journal of Allergy and Clinical Immunology*, 130: 427–434.

Pericone, C. D., Overweg, K., Hermans, P. W. M., Weiser J. N. (2000) 'Inhibitory and bactericidal effects of hydrogen peroxide production by streptococcus pneumoniae on other inhabitants of the upper respiratory tract,' *Infection and Immunity*, 68: 3990–3997.

Lysenko, E. S., Ratner, A. J., Nelson, A. L., and Weiser, J. N. (2005) 'The role of innate immune responses in the outcome of interspecies competition for colonization of mucosal surfaces,' *PLoS Pathogens*, 1(1): e1.

Tapiainen, T., Sormunen, R., Kaijalainen, T., Kontiokari, T., Ikäheimo, I., Uhari, M. (2004) 'Ultrastructure of streptococcus pneumoniae after exposure to xylitol', *Journal of Antimicrobial Chemotherapy*, 54: 225–228.

Matthews S. B., Waud J. P., Roberts A. G., et al. (2005) 'Systemic lactose intolerance: A new perspective on an old problem,' *Postgraduate Medical Journal*, 81: 167–173.

Gevorgyan A., Segboer C., Gorissen R., van Drunen C. M., Fokkens W. (2015) 'Capsaicin for non-allergic rhinitis,' *Cochrane Database of Systematic Reviews*, Issue 7. Art. No.: CD010591. DOI:10.1002/14651858. CD010591.pub2.

CHAPTER 4

Truelsen, T., Nielsen, N., Boysen, G., and Grønbæk, M. (2003) 'Self-reported stress and risk of stroke: The Copenhagen city heart study,' *Stroke*, 234: 856–862.

Booth, J., Connelly, L., Lawrence, M. et al. (2015) 'Evidence of perceived psychosocial stress as a risk factor for stroke in adults: a meta-analysis,' *BMC Neurol*, 15: 233. https://DOI.org/10.1186/s12883-015-0456-4.

Tawakol, A., Ishai, A., Takx, R. A. P., Figueroa, A. L., Ali, A., Kaiser, Y., Truong, Q. A., Solomon, C. J. E., Calcagno, C., Mani, V., Tang, C. Y., Mulder, W. J. M., Murrough, J. W., Hoffmann, U., Nahrendorf, M., Shin, L. M., Fayad, Z. A., Pitman, R. K. (2017) 'Relation between resting amygdalar activity and cardiovascular events: A longitudinal and cohort study,' *The Lancet*, 389(10071): 834–845.

Lazar, S. W., Bush, G., Gollub, R. L., Fricchione, G. L., Khalsa, G., Benson, H. (2000) 'Functional brain mapping of the relaxation response and meditation,' *NeuroReport*, 11(7): 1581–1585.

Mischkowski, D., Crocker, J., Way, B. M. (2016) 'From painkiller to empathy killer: acetaminophen (paracetamol) reduces empathy for pain,' *Social Cognitive and Affective Neuroscience*, 11(9): 1345–1353. https://doi.org/10.1093/scan/nsw057.

CHAPTER 5

Barson J. R., Leibowitz, S. F. (2017) 'Orexin/hypocretin system: role in food and drug overconsumption,' *International Review of Neurobiology*, 136: 199–237.

Ferrari, A., Zappaterra, M., Righi, F. et al. (2013) 'Impact of continuing or quitting smoking on episodic cluster headache: A pilot survey,' *J. Headache Pain*, 14: 48. https://doi.org/10.1186/1129-2377-14-48.

Horton, B. T. (1961) 'Histaminic cephalgia (Horton's headache or syndrome),' *Maryland State Medical Journal*, 10: 178–203.

Nicolodi, M., Sicuteri, F. and Poggioni, M. (1993), 'Hypothalamic modulation of nociception and reproduction in cluster headache, II. Testosterone-induced increase of sexual activity in males with cluster headache,' *Cephalalgia*, 13: 258–260. DOI:10.1046/j.1468-2982.1993.1304258.x.

Fanciullacci, M. (2006) 'When cluster headache was called histaminic cephalalgia (Horton's headache),' *J. Headache Pain*, 7: 231–234. https://doi.org/10.1007/s10194-006-0296-0.

May, A., Bahra, A., Büchel, C., Frackowiak, R. S. J, Goadsby, P. J. (1998) 'Hypothalamic activation in cluster headache attacks,' *The Lancet*, 352(9124): 275–278.

Naegel, S., Holle, D., Desmarattes, N., Theysohn, N., Diener, H.-C., Katsarava, Z., Obermann, M. (2014) 'Cortical plasticity in episodic and chronic cluster headache,' *NeuroImage: Clinical*, 6: 415–423.

Akerman, S., Holland, P. R., Lasalandra, M. P. and Goadsby, P. J. (2009) 'Oxygen inhibits neuronal activation in the trigeminocervical complex after stimulation of trigeminal autonomic reflex, but not during direct dural activation of trigeminal afferents,' *Headache: The Journal of Head and Face Pain*, 49: 1131–1143. DOI:10.1111/j.1526-4610.2009.01501.x.

Gotkine M., Steiner I., Biran I. (2006) 'Now dear, I have a headache! Immediate improvement of cluster headaches after sexual activity,' *Journal of Neurology, Neurosurgery & Psychiatry*, 77: 1296.

CHAPTER 6

Gago-Veiga, A. B., Pagán, J., Henares, K., Heredia, P., González-García, N., De Orbe, M. I., Ayala, J. L., Sobrado, M., and Vivancos, J. (2018), 'To what extent are patients with migraine able to predict attacks?' *Journal of Pain Research*, 11: 2083–2094. https://doi.org/10.2147/JPR.S175602.

Gallup, A. C., Gallup, Gordon G. (2008) 'Yawning and thermoregulation,' *Physiology & Behavior*, 95: 10–16.

Barbanti, P., Fofi, L., Aurilia, C. et al. (2013) 'Dopaminergic symptoms in migraine,' Neurol Sci, 34: 67–70. https://doi.org/10.1007/s10072-013-1415-8.

Penfield, W., and Rasmussen, T. (1950) *The Cerebral Cortex of Man: A Clinical Study of Localization of Function*. (London: Macmillan).

Lashley K. S. (1941) 'Patterns of cerebral integration indicated by the scotomas of migraine,' *Arch Neurol Psych.*, 46: 331–339.

Gowers W. R. (1906). Clinical Lectures on the borderland of epilepsy. III Migraine. *BMJ*, 2(2397): 1617–1622. https://doi.org/10.1136/bmj.2.2397.1617.

Barkley, G., Tepley, N., Nagel-Leiby, S., Moran, J., Simkins, R. and Welch, K. (1990) 'Magnetoencephalographic studies of migraine,' *Headache: The Journal of Head and Face Pain*, 30: 428–434. DOI:10.1111/j.1526-4610.1990.hed3007428.x.

Barratt E. L., Spence C., Davis N. J. (2017) 'Sensory determinants of the autonomous sensory meridian response (ASMR): understanding the triggers,' *PeerJ* 5:e3846. https://doi.org/10.7717/peerj.3846.

Goadsby, P. J. (2001) 'Migraine, aura, and cortical spreading depression: why are we still talking about it?' *Ann Neurol.*, 49: 4–6. DOI:10.1002/1531-8249(200101)49:1<4::AID-ANA3>3.0.CO;2-W.

Harriott, A. M., Takizawa, T., Chung, D. Y. et al. (2019) 'Spreading depression as a preclinical model of migraine,' *J Headache Pain* 20(45). https://doi.org/10.1186/s10194-019-1001-4.

CHAPTER 7

Selinsky H. (1939) 'Psychological Study of the Migrainous Syndrome,' *Bulletin of the New York Academy of Medicine*, 15(11), 757–763.

Wray, S. H., Mijović-Prelec, D., Kosslyn, S. M. (1995) 'Visual processing in migraineurs,' *Brain*, 118(1) 25–35. https://doi.org/10.1093/brain/118.1.25.

Mulleners, W. M., Chronicle, E. P., Palmer, J. E., Koehler, P. J. and Vredeveld, J.-W. (2001) 'Visual cortex excitability in migraine with and without aura,' *Headache: The Journal of Head and Face Pain*, 41: 565–572. DOI:10.1046/j.1526-4610.2001.041006565.x.

Hagen, K., Åsvold, B. O., Midthjell, K., Stovner, L. J., Zwart, J.-A. (2017) 'Inverse relationship between type 1 diabetes mellitus and migraine,' Data from the Nord-Trøndelag Health Surveys 1995–1997 and 2006–2008. *Cephalgia*, 38: 417–426.

Goadsby, P. J. (2008) 'Calcitonin gene-related peptide (CGRP) antagonists and migraine,' *Neurology*, 70(16): 1300–1301. DOI:10.1212/01.wnl.0000309214.25038.fd.

Houle, T. T., Dhingra, L. K., Remble, T. A., Rokicki, L. A. and Penzien, D. B. (2006) 'Not tonight, I have a headache?' *Headache: The Journal of Head and Face Pain*, 46: 983–990. DOI:10.1111/j.1526-4610.2006.00470.x.

Ferrero S., Pretta S., Bertoldi S., Anserini P., Remorgida V., et al. (2004) 'Increased frequency of migraine among women with endometriosis,' *Hum Reprod.* 19: 2927–2932.

Hausmann, M. (2005) 'Hemispheric asymmetry in spatial attention across the menstrual cycle,' *Neuropsychologia*, 43: 1559–1567.

Schwerzmann, M., Nedeltchev, K., Lagger, F., Mattle, H. P., Windecker, S., Meier, B., Seiler, C. (2005) 'Prevalence and size of directly detected patent foramen ovale in migraine with aura,' *Neurology*, 65: 1415–1418.

Mullen, M. J., Devellian, C. A. and Jux, C. (2007) 'BioSTAR® bioabsorbable septal repair implant', *Expert Review of Medical Devices*, 4(6): 781–792. DOI:10.1586/17434440.4.6.781.

Turner, D. P., Smitherman, T. A., Penzien, D. B., Porter, J. A. H., Martin, V. T., Houle, T. T. (2014) 'Nighttime snacking, stress, and migraine activity,' *Journal of Clinical Neuroscience*, 21: 638–643.

Kwok, R. H. M. (1968) 'Chinese-Restaurant Syndrome,' *N Engl J Med*, 278: 796. DOI: 10.1056/NEJM196804042781419.

Schaumburg, H. H., Byck, R., Gerstl, R., Mashman, J. H. (1969) 'Monosodium L-Glutamate: its pharmacology and role in the Chinese restaurant syndrome,' *Science*, 21: 826–828.

Gonzalez, A., Hyde, E., Sangwan, N., Gilbert, J. A., Viirre, E., Knight, R. (2016) 'Migraines are correlated with higher levels of nitrate-, nitrite-, and nitric oxide-reducing oral microbes in the American Gut Project cohort,' *mSystems*, 1(5): e00105–16. DOI:10.1128/mSystems.00105-16.

Kapil, V., Haydar, S. M. A., Pearl, V., Lundberg, J. O., Weitzberg, E., Ahluwalia, A. (2013) 'Physiological role for nitrate-reducing oral bacteria in blood pressure control,' *Free Radical Biology and Medicine*, 55: 93–100.

Chapter 8

Llinás, R. R., Ribary, U., Jeanmonod, D., Kronberg, E., Mitra, P. P. (1999) 'Thalamocortical dysrhythmia: a neurological and neuropsychiatric syndrome characterized by magnetoencephalography,' *Proceedings of the National Academy of Sciences*, 96: 15222–15227. DOI:10.1073/pnas.96.26.15222.

Jeanmonod, D., Magnin, M., Morel, A., Siegemund, M., Cancro, A., Lanz, M., . . . Zonenshayn, M. (2001) 'Thalamocortical dysrhythmia II. Clinical and surgical aspects,' *Thalamus & Related Systems*, 1(3): 245–254. DOI:10.1017/S1472928801000267.

Akram, H., Miller, S., Lagrata, S., Hariz, M., Ashburner, J., Behrens, T., Matharu, M., Zrinzo, L. (2017) 'Optimal deep brain stimulation site and target connectivity for chronic cluster headache,' *Neurology*, 89: 2083–2091. DOI:10.1212/WNL.0000000000004646.

Labots, G., Jones, A., de Visser, S. J., Rissmann, R., and Burggraaf, J. (2018) 'Gender differences in clinical registration trials: is there a real problem?' *Br J Clin Pharmacol*, 84: 700–707. DOI:10.1111/bcp.13497.

Messinger, H., Messinger, M., Kudrow, L. and Kudrow, L. (1994) 'Handedness and headache,' *Cephalalgia*, 14: 64–67. DOI:10.1046/j.1468-2982.1994.1401064.x.

Index

INDEX

oral contraceptives 178
orexin/hypocretin 95–7, 102, 118–20
oxygen 3, 67, 69, 70, 75–6, 97, 107, 115, 116
oxytocin 80, 121–2

pain gating 48
pain threshold 8, 146, 147
painkillers 5, 7–8, 58, 85, 86–8
paracetamol 5, 7, 58, 85, 86–8, 196
parasympathetic 'rest-and-digest' nervous system 30, 66, 102, 107
parenting 79–80
parietal cortex 4, 146
parietal lobe 87, 137
Parkinson's disease 116, 201–3
patent foramen ovale 179–83
pet dander 42, 51
petrous temporal bones 22
phenols 195–6
phosphenes 124–5, 170
photic sneezing 29–30
photophobia 146, 169
pituitary gland 66, 67–8, 175
pollen 34–5, 42, 57
potassium 139–41
see also ion balance and nerve cells
preoptic nucleus 100, 110
proprioception 128
prostaglandins 2, 28, 87, 141, 177
protein production 93–4, 95, 158
PST-P 195–6
puberty 45, 100
pupillary responses 102

questionnaires, health 45–7

rapid eye movement sleep (REM) 99
referred pain 18–19, 145
resilience, stress and 81–2
rhinitis 28, 44
rhinorrhoea 40
rhinovirus 35

scans, CT 50
scotoma 123, 125–6
Seasonal Affective Disorder (SAD) 98–9
selective serotonin-reuptake inhibitors (SSRIs) 175
sensory auras, non-visual 126–8
serotonin 7, 77, 79, 85, 88, 89, 98, 102, 108–9, 110, 111, 118, 120–1, 167–8, 174–5, 194

sex 30, 100–1, 111, 122, 174
sinus anatomy and physiology 21, 27, 33–5, 44–5
sinusitis
    allergies 33–5, 41–4, 51, 58
    bacteria and viruses 35–9, 52–3
    cross-diagnosis 28–9, 48–9, 60
    histamine 26, 28, 29, 34–5, 41, 57
    impact on day-to-day life 45–9
    internal causes 44–5
    investigating 49–51
    irritants 39–41, 51
    mucus/snot 23–5, 28, 29, 33, 40, 50
    pain in your face 27
    swimming pools etc 31–3
    sneezing 29–30
    surgical solutions 53–4
    symptoms overview 21–3
    treating 51–60
skin hypersensitivity 126–7
sleep 3, 47, 72, 99, 120, 148
smoking 96
sneezing 29–30
snot 23–5
see also mucus
SNOT-22 questionnaire 46–7
somatosensation 128
somatosensory auras 127
somatosensory cortex 137, 146, 147
sphenoid sinuses 21, 27, 44, 48
sphenopalatine ganglion 17
spicy food 39–40
spinal trigeminal nucleus 145
spreading oligaemia 140–1
steroids 57–8
stomach ulcers 101–2
Streptococcus pneumonia 36, 37–8, 39
stress 3, 56, 61–2, 63–8, 74–5, 79–86
stress headaches *see* tension headaches
strokes 69–70, 162, 181
subarachnoid haemorrhage 6
sulphites 194
sumatriptan 107–9, 174, 197, 206
suprachiasmatic nucleus (SCN) 98–100, 102, 104
surfer's skull 16
swimming pools 31–2
sympathetic 'fight-or-flight' nervous system 66–7, 68, 70–1, 76, 78, 82, 84, 102
symptom diaries 49, 210
synapses 134–5

temporal cortex 4, 146
temporal lobe 104, 136
tension headaches 48–9, 60, 62–3
    adrenaline as trigger 69
    autonomic nervous system 66–7
    building resilience 80–2
    classical conditioning 84
    cyclical nature of 72–6
    dehydration 75–6
    emotions 64–6, 74, 81, 82–4
    endocrine system 67–8
    food and drink 75, 76–8
    immersion therapy 89
    immune response 69–70
    medications 82, 85–8
    meditation 82–4
    musculature 71, 73
    nitric oxide (NO) 71
    posture 73–4, 79, 89
    responding to stress 79–84
testosterone 100–1, 102
Thalamocortical Dysrhythmia 203–4
thalamus 145–6, 202–4
transcranial magnetic stimulation (TMS) 124, 170, 201, 204–5
transcutaneous vagal nerve stimulation (tVNS) 206
trephination 144
trigeminal nerve and pathway 18–19, 29–30, 70, 71, 103, 107, 120, 122, 141, 142, 145, 146, 177, 206
tryptophan 121
tyramine 185–6, 195

underactive thyroid 45

vagus nerve 206
vasoconstrictors 106, 111, 120, 140, 148, 174, 194
vasodilation 4, 41, 71, 75–6, 78, 97, 103, 110, 111, 141, 142, 143, 168, 174, 181, 184, 191–2, 194
Verapamil 110
viruses 31, 35–6, 54
visual cortex 4, 125–6, 135, 146, 168–72
vitamin D 98–9

warfarin 182
water 8–9
waves of excitation 128–35, 137–9, 203
white blood cells 26, 35, 57, 70

yawning 115–18

zona incerta 87, 146–7

233

Acknowledgements

There are many people to thank for their support in the publishing of this book but my first point of thanks is more existential. Without Jaime Marshall, my agent, it would not have been born. The day I answered your phone call, Jaime, was an excellent day on the planet. I considerably enjoy our conversations and much appreciate your sage guidance. You are my own personal lightbulb! Huge thanks to my editors, Charlotte Croft and Zoë Blanc, for your tireless efforts to make this book better and your enthusiasm about the project in general and to Jasmine Parker for her lovely illustrations. My correspondents have been invaluable. In addition to all the people who have shared their experience of headache with me (I hope you see yourself in these pages), specific thanks to Kate Blackmore, Maya Kaczorowski, Jennifer Crampton and all the academics and health professionals whose ears I chewed during the writing of this book. Lastly, thanks to my family. You all know why.